The Mindful Nurse

Using the Power of Mindfulness and Compassion to Help You Thrive in Your Work

Praise for *The Mindful Nurse:*

This book should be a part of every nurse's education. As healthcare providers, we need to know ourselves and that we have needs, too. These needs can be met through mindfulness and compassion so that not curing a disease does not make us failures.

Bernie Siegel, MD
Author of *A Book of Miracles* and *The Art of Healing*

Every staff nurse reading this book will say, "YES! This is nursing!" Every nurse often asks the question, "How can I manage that situation better?" Within the wisdom of this book are solutions. The suggested self-care, guidance, and techniques will raise the quality of nursing care and patient satisfaction.

Carole Ann Drick, PhD, RN, AHN-BC
President, American Holistic Nurses Association,
Author of *End of Life: Nursing Solutions for Death with Dignity*

Mindfulness is all the rage right now, and if you do not understand it and don't know what it can do for you and your personal and professional life, then this book will help. It guides you through the who, what, why, and how of the practice of mindfulness—all through the eyes of an author who relates it to nurses' everyday lives and tasks. Carmel shows how it can improve your own life and the care you give to patients. The turns of phrase and concepts supporting the practice of mindfulness are delicious—I most loved the idea that self-compassion was an "antiseptic" and "anti-inflammatory" for those moments when you beat yourself up or blame others when things go wrong. There are lots of practical elements to help you start practicing mindfulness, from the moment you pick up the book, to encourage you to make mindfulness a daily part of your life so that you can enjoy living more.

Jenni Middleton
Editor, *Nursing Times*

Carmel brings her experience of working with healthcare professionals together with her understanding of mindfulness practice to share a wealth of practical resources. All this is in service of supporting nurses to develop essential self-care skills. The result is a book that could make a great contribution to nursing school curricula around the globe.

Sharon Salzberg,
Author of *Lovingkindness* and *Real Happiness*

An incredibly valuable tool for all nurses, whether beginning their career, reaching the point of burnout, or somewhere in between. If you are wondering where your love of the job has gone, here are achievable exercises to reconnect with that. The love is still potentially there but often lost under the stress and exhaustion that is all too common in the nursing profession. This book offers practical tools for nurses who want to serve but also to nurture themselves.

Bronnie Ware
Author of *The Top Five Regrets of the Dying*

This excellent book provides a guide for nurses and health care providers on how to incorporate mindfulness practices into their work routine and everyday life. Written in a very engaging and accessible style, it offers practical guidance on applying a range of very feasible yet powerful practices that can enhance mental health and wellbeing and reduce stress and burnout. This is a very valuable addition to the current literature on mindfulness training and health promotion in the workplace.

Margaret M. Barry, PhD
Professor of Health Promotion and Public Health,
World Health Organization Collaborating Centre for Health
Promotion Research, NUI Galway, Ireland.

Drawing on recent groundbreaking research in the field of neuroscience, Sheridan offers an extremely readable and insightful guidebook to help nurses cultivate resilience and therapeutic presence and revitalize their practice. An excellent resource for nurses in both clinical and educational settings.

Janice M Zeller, PhD, RN, FAAN
Professor and Graduate Program Director,
North Park University School of Nursing

A much-needed, well written, and full-of-wisdom guide to help care for the caregiver. Nurses and other healing professionals will benefit immensely from these clear and helpful mindfulness tools and practices. I imagine a quiet revolution in hospitals as nurses begin to embody mindfulness and compassion, transforming their own lives and the lives of everyone they touch.

Diana Winston
Director of Mindfulness Education,
UCLA Mindful Awareness Research Center
Author of *Fully Present: The Science, Art, and Practice of Mindfulness*

This book offers hardworking nurses a path forward. Finally, there is an accessible and effective way to avoid burnout and become healthy, balanced, and grounded. An invaluable resource!

Barbara Dossey, PhD, RN, FAAN
Author of *Nurse Coaching: Integrative Approaches for Health and Wellbeing; Holistic Nursing: A Handbook for Practice*; and *Florence Nightingale: Mystic, Visionary, Healer*

This is a book to which all nurses can relate…an easy read, but with very deep and life-altering content. Guard this book with your (mindful) life!

Kimberly Kimbrough BSN, RN
24 year Renal Dialysis/transplant nurse
Nashville, TN

Being more mindful may help practicing nurses and students of nursing enhance their professional practice as well as prevent burnout. Learning how to better care for oneself and one's patients is what Carmel offers in this much-needed and practical guide for nurses wishing to develop greater mindfulness in their practice and personal lives.

Lois Howland, PhD, MSN, RN
Associate Professor, Hahn School of Nursing and Health Science, University of California San Diego;
Senior Teacher, Center for Mindfulness, UCSD

The Mindful Nurse

Using the Power of Mindfulness and Compassion to Help You Thrive in Your Work

By Carmel Sheridan

Rivertime Press

Rivertime Press
©2016 by Rivertime Press

www.rivertimepress.com
Printed in the United States of America

The information in this book is not intended as a substitute for medical treatment or advice.

Library of Congress Cataloging-in-Publication Data
Sheridan, Carmel B
The Mindful Nurse: Using the Power of Mindfulness and Compassion to Help You Thrive in Your Work
1st ed.
Includes bibliographical references and index

ISBN 978-0-9933245-2-9 (paperback)
ISBN 978-0-9933245-3-6 (ebook)

Library of Congress Control Number: 2016950636

British Library Cataloguing-in-Publication Data
A CIP record for this book is available from the British Library.

For information about custom editions of this book and special discounts for bulk purchases, please contact Rivertime Special Sales Department at specialsales@rivertimepress.com or 800-280-9679

This book is dedicated to nurses everywhere.
May the practices of mindfulness
and compassion enrich your work
and benefit those in your care.

To enter fully the day, the hour, the moment—whether it appears as life or death, whether we catch it on the inbreath or outbreath— requires only a moment, this moment.

—Stephen Levine

Contents

Preface 13

Acknowledgements 15

Introduction 17

PART I
Embracing Mindfulness

Chapter 1: What Is Mindfulness? 25
Chapter 2: Doing and Being 45
Chapter 3: Everyday Mindfulness 57
Chapter 4: Reaping the Benefits of Mindfulness Practice...... 73

PART II
Mindfulness and the Body

Chapter 5: Mindful Self-Care 89
Chapter 6: Inhabiting Your Body 103
Chapter 7: Preventing Injury the Mindful Way 125
Chapter 8: Coping Mindfully with Pain 135
Chapter 9: Coping with Stress the Mindful Way 143
Chapter 10: Mindful Movement 157

PART III
Compassion—The Essence of Mindfulness

Chapter 11: Understanding Compassion 173
Chapter 12: The Constant Giver: Compassion Fatigue 187
Chapter 13: Cultivating Self-Compassion 199
Chapter 14: Strengthening Compassion 213

PART IV
Mindfulness For Better Performance

Chapter 15: Working with Thoughts 235
Chapter 16: Mindful Teamwork...249
Chapter 17: Mindful Communication 259
Chapter 18: Working with Distractions,
    Preventing Errors 271
Chapter 19: The Mindful Handover Report 287
Chapter 20: The Challenge of Advancing Technology 297
Chapter 21: Bringing Mindfulness and Compassion
    to your Healthcare Facility 307

Moving Forward Mindfully..323

Appendix A: List Of Practices 325

Appendix B: ProQOL 327

Additional Resources (by Chapter) 331

Notes..338

References 347

Index..367

About the Author..372

Preface

Each person is unique, but in my years of practice as a psychotherapist, I have seen certain characteristics shared by those in the helping professions, including compassion, understanding, drive, stress, and fatigue. Those who help others often face the double-edged sword of giving their resources to others while depleting their own.

Many of the health professionals whom I see in private practice are nurses spanning every specialty. From critical care to oncology, and emergency nurses, I have assisted many of these dedicated caregivers through the stresses of compassion fatigue, depression, substance abuse, poor boundary setting, and neglected self-care, all of which arise from giving so much of themselves to others.

Often, nurses and other healthcare providers are the "invisible patients." The focus of care is always on their assigned patients, but what about the health of the nurses themselves? How is their mental health? When is the last time they had a good night's sleep? When is the last time they spent quality time with their family? Regrettably, their own needs are often ignored or pushed to the back burner.

Mindfulness offers a solution. In teaching nurses to cultivate mindfulness and compassion, I have witnessed how these practices can dramatically reduce their stress and fatigue. Nurses who integrate these practices into their lives make lasting improvements in how they respond to everyday stress and avoid burnout. These nurses get their energy back. They learn to be fully present with themselves and their patients, often restoring their love of the profession.

Mindfulness and compassion practices are de-stressors, antidotes to the pervasive pressures you experience on a daily basis. They will help you to stay resilient, focused, present, and compassionate, not just with your patients but—as importantly—with yourself.

This book was written specifically for you, the nurse, to address your particular concerns and specific needs. By focusing on where you can make a difference—in the present, here and now—and extending to yourself the same quality of care and compassion that you extend to others, you can energize yourself, enliven your work, and turn things around if burnout has depleted you.

It is my goal to inspire you to explore new ways of being fully present with yourself and the people whose lives you touch, helping you to thrive in your work and live your vision fully.

Acknowledgments

I would like to thank the teachers who have helped me understand mindfulness over the years. These include Jack Kornfield and the teachers at Spirit Rock Meditation Center in Woodacre, California, where I first began my mindfulness journey in the early '90s.

I'm grateful to the teachers at the Center for Mindfulness, Health Care, and Society at UMass who introduced me to Mindfulness-Based Stress Reduction (MBSR). Specifically, I would like to thank Jon Kabat-Zinn, Saki Santorelli, Florence Meleo-Meyer, and Melissa Blacker. Their integrity and heartfulness have been an inspiration to me.

For their pioneering work in compassion and self-compassion, much of which is discussed in this book, I'm grateful to Paul Gilbert, Kristin Neff, and Chris Germer.

My thanks to the nurses who have attended my mindfulness trainings and psychotherapy practice over the years. Their struggles with staying present, openhearted, and well in our busy, stressed healthcare system sowed the seeds for this book.

Thanks to editor Donna Magnani for her attentive and insightful edits on early iterations of this book.

I would also like to thank librarian Siobhan Carroll at Nursing & Midwifery Library, James Hardiman Library, National University of Ireland, Galway, for her generous help in tracking down useful resources.

I am grateful to Patricia Suresh, Audit and Practice Development Facilitator at Our Lady of Lourdes Hospital in Drogheda, for information relating to the Nursing Stress Scale.

I appreciate everyone (especially Gearoid) at Esker Redemptorists' Retreat Center, Co. Galway, Ireland, for opening their doors to mindfulness and allowing me a beautiful venue for teaching.

A sincere thank-you to my friends, who patiently accepted my long absences and preoccupied mind while I worked on this book.

Huge appreciation to my son Jamie, for bringing me so much happiness. May your life blossom!

Finally, my thanks to Cahal, whose unwavering patience sustained me during many months of writing. I am grateful for your kind and mindful presence in my life.

May you all be well.

Introduction

*The most precious gift we can offer others is our presence. When
mindfulness embraces those we love, they will bloom like flowers.*

—Thich Nhat Hanh

You have just walked out of report to start your first shift. Several
patients already have their call lights on, and family members are
trying to get your attention. People are rushing around, and you have
a hard time prioritizing what to do first.

You make a quick decision and dive in, answering a call light
to take a patient to the bathroom. By the time you're done, four
other lights are flashing and the floor is even more hectic. You dive
in again, answering call after call, working hard to tend to all your
patients' needs.

While you pass out medications, a colleague arrives to report that
one of your patients has a blood pressure reading of 220/110. The
meds will have to wait. You jog across the hall to assess your patient
and plan the appropriate intervention.

The situation takes hours to resolve. During this time, you have
doctors to call and vitals to take, not to mention a multitude of other
things to do. You work and work and work, taking no time to tend to
your own needs. By the end of your shift, you are exhausted.

Sound familiar? As a nurse, you are a crucial link in the medical
chain. You are the oil that keeps the great medical machinery
running. You are the coordinator, the caregiver, the frontline referee.
You are also expected to be the human face of healthcare: unfaltering,
dedicated, and with unlimited reserves of compassion and empathy.
The rewards of your profession come at a price. You put in long
hours, meet impossible demands, and deal with a high level of stress.

Many nurses know they should tend to their own needs, yet they continue to put self-care on the back burner. This is common behavior for today's busy nurses. Does this sound like you? Even while you advise patients on their eating and exercise habits, their smoking and drinking, and even after you teach them how to de-stress, you ignore your own unhealthy lifestyle. You ignore your aching feet, sore back, and tension headache. You don't work out and often stuff yourself with unhealthy food during rushed coffee breaks. Worse yet, you may skip meals and breaks altogether. Maybe you even sneak a cigarette after work or drink a few too many glasses of wine.

Nursing is a demanding profession. Sometimes the unmitigated chaos can result not only in exhaustion but also in the career killer: burnout. It is not surprising that many nurses abandon the field: they are mentally and physically exhausted. They just can't do it anymore.

But this does not have to happen to you. This book will show how mindfulness and compassion can help you practice nursing in a way that allows you to also care for yourself, and avoid burning out.

What to Expect

The following are just a few of the things you will learn:

- Mindfulness and Compassion Practices: To help you better manage stress, pay attention, and cultivate compassion with specific practices including the body scan, as well as eating-, sitting-, walking-, and loving-kindness meditations.
- Awareness: To better recognize when your mind slips into "autopilot" mode so you can gently bring yourself back to awareness.
- Peaceful Moments: To find new ways to create little islands of peace in the rush and bustle of your everyday life as a nurse.
- Becoming Present: To help you tune in rather than tune out so you can listen attentively and communicate better, strengthening your relationships with self, patients, colleagues, and others.

🍃 Balancing Doing and Being: To develop a healthy balance between doing and being to help improve your personal well-being and work productivity.

What Mindfulness Can Do

Although the stress inherent in nursing may seem inescapable, you *can* change things for the better. It requires learning a new skill, one that may seem simpler than CPR or changing an occupied bed, but you need to train yourself to use it, just as you trained yourself to use all of your nursing skills. That skill is mindfulness and, fortunately, it is a skill you can learn and cultivate.

Mindfulness is a way of being that promotes a return to the present moment; its practice cultivates awareness. It is also a self-care practice to help you avoid that slippery slope into burnout, strengthening your ability to slow down, concentrate, and pay attention to what matters most. Scientifically proven to have many health benefits, mindfulness anchors you in the present moment, freeing your busy mind to focus on the here and now. Although it requires persistence and patience, mindfulness is an investment well worth your time. With regular practice, you'll see changes in your attitude toward work, your relationships, and even your lifestyle.

Developing mindfulness is a process of learning to bring a new way of being into daily life, helping you to cope even in situations when you are under pressure, which is often the case in nursing. According to Susan Bauer-Wu, Director of the Compassionate Care Initiative at the University of Virginia School of Nursing, nurses in the future will receive mindfulness training just as they now learn to insert an IV or assess pain.[1] Why wait for "the future" when you can make these positive changes in your life right now?

Compassion and Self-Compassion

Cultivating compassion in the healthcare facility is equally important. In healthcare, people skills matter most. A nurse's kind words go a long way in helping patients feel supported. Likewise, patients will remember a doctor's bedside manner long after the illness is cured and forgotten. Patients look for these qualities in a healthcare facility because, when they are sick, they want to be treated with kindness and compassion.

Although nurses are blessed with naturally strong "compassion muscles," unfortunately, these muscles are subject to fatigue and injury. Challenging work environments, short-staffing, increased patient numbers and acuity, as well as repeated exposure to the suffering of others can challenge your natural instinct to feel and show compassion. Compassion fatigue is a well-known phenomenon in the nursing profession. When it strikes, you may show signs of emotional exhaustion and become less effective at work. If not addressed early, these symptoms may spiral into full-blown compassion fatigue and lead to burnout over time.

As a nurse, you do the heavy lifting in ensuring your patients and their families feel cared for, comforted, and hopeful. Day in and day out, you actively soothe and care for people during their most vulnerable, fear-filled, and painful moments. With so many critical demands placed on you in the workplace, you tend to put your own needs aside in order to do your job. Long work hours and additional responsibilities, such as your spouse, children, or parent, can convince you that, no matter what, there is never enough time in your day. The smallest things—like a pile of dirty laundry or a missed dinner date—can lead to intense self-criticism, and a mistake at work can lead to dire consequences, fueling in you a heightened vigilance for even the smallest of errors.

In the end, beating yourself up, or blaming others, only makes things worse. It's a bit like putting a dirty bandage on a fresh wound and expecting it to heal properly. The antidote lies in deliberately training in compassion. Think of self-compassion as the antiseptic and anti-inflammatory for these moments. Compassion for your own vulnerability and humanity can cleanse you of any toxic emotions and soothe that harsh self-criticism.

Self-compassion is the ability to comfort yourself by converting feelings of blame and shame into acceptance and kindness. A skill and a practice, self-compassion means becoming your own best friend. It must be built up just like a muscle in the body that, with training, becomes stronger and more resilient. This book will show you how to grow in compassion by first turning it inward, toward yourself.

As you practice these skills, you'll discover that distraction, mindlessness, and criticism occur less often, making way for compassion and self-care. Your ability to solve problems in stressful situations will improve, boosting your confidence and efficiency. Eventually, you may also become a better team player at work, and a more supportive family member at home, because you'll be better able to accept other people's faults or mistakes and to notice opportunities to provide support and kindness.

In my work as a psychotherapist helping healthcare professionals over the years, I've met many nurses who have overextended themselves in the demanding, turbulent medical environment. And I've witnessed how the practices of mindfulness and compassion can rejuvenate the spirit and restore the nurse's ability to be wholehearted at work. Time and again I have seen nurses learn to draw on their own inner wellspring of peace, and cope with stress in new ways without the emotional toll of burnout.

Throughout the book you will read real-life anecdotes about nurses who have struggled with issues faced by most nurses during their career. You will discover the benefits these practices have had in their careers and in their personal lives.

It takes time to make mindfulness a habit—just as it takes time to make anything a habit—but once you do, you will cope with stress in a healthier way and feel calmer. Imagine no longer flitting from one thought to the next and wasting your precious emotional resources on worry and self-criticism.

Ready to get started?

How to Use This Book

Before you embark on this journey, consider keeping a notebook or journal to record and reflect on your experiences of the practices introduced in this book. *Journal Reflection* sections have been added throughout the book to encourage you to record your experiences. Bear in mind that mindfulness is called a practice because it has to be practiced regularly. As you try out the practices and repeat them daily, note your experiences in the journal. Although you may read through the whole book without doing this, you will benefit far more by pausing at intervals to fully integrate the practices explored so far and record your experiences. You might consider giving yourself a week to work through each chapter, establishing a daily practice as you go. Don't worry—not every chapter will take a week. The idea is simply to give yourself time to absorb the teachings and incorporate the practices into your daily routine.

Take advantage of the *Practice Plan* in each chapter as a suggestion for your weekly focus, and be sure to check *Additional Resources* for each chapter, provided near the end of the book. See Appendix A for a list of all the practices described in this book. Also take a moment to visit www.nursingmindfully.com, where many practices you'll learn about in your reading are available as free downloads in either audio or video format.

Remember, you can talk about mindfulness or read about it, but the real benefit comes from putting it into practice and experiencing it directly. So notice any impulse you have to power through the chapters until you reach the finish line. Instead, take your time to discover for yourself how these practices can enrich your everyday life and work.

PART I
EMBRACING MINDFULNESS

Few of us ever live in the present. We are forever anticipating what is to come or remembering what has gone.

—Louis L'Amour

CHAPTER ONE

What Is Mindfulness?

Our duty is wakefulness, the fundamental condition of life itself.
—Robin Craig Clark

Stephanie loved working at the bedside and, as a floor nurse, enjoyed the challenge of facing something new on the floor every day, yet she struggled to remember her patients' details as well as their lab values and medications.

One moment her mind would be on charting, and the next moment, as she stood in front of the medication dispenser, she would be thinking of the wound change that needed attention in room five. Then, as she administered the medication, the phone would ring and a doctor would be on the other end. While listening to the doctor's orders, Stephanie would worry about the patient whose call light was on. As a result, the doctor would have to repeat the orders three times, as Stephanie was not paying full attention.

As she sat at a computer, charting after her shift, Stephanie would go over the day's work in her head, searching for anything she missed. It didn't let up as she drove home. Instead of focusing on her driving, she would be thinking about that IV she couldn't get started. Once Stephanie was so distracted that she ran a stop sign. No one was around, but it was scary to think she could have hurt someone.

Monkey Mind
Like Stephanie, many nurses suffer from "monkey mind." Like a restless monkey swinging from one tree branch to another, their minds leap from one thought to the next.

Rather than focusing on each situation as it happens, monkey mind sends your thoughts spinning with distractions, leading to stress and emotional overwhelm. You worry about problems that might occur as a shift progresses or problems that have already happened, as well as the multitude of things that remain to be done. Juggling so many things, your mind is usually two steps ahead, always on, but rarely present.

Consider This:

How often do you mentally rehash difficult conversations you've had? Perhaps one with a patient's family, struggling with their loved one's illness?

Do you regularly obsess about getting all your charting done?

Do you repeatedly replay criticism from coworkers?

What about when taking care of a patient whose condition is deteriorating? Do you ruminate endlessly on the plights of others?

Such distressing thoughts not only distract you from what is going on inside and around you but can also make you feel stressed and tired.

As a nurse, you are often bombarded with demands on your time throughout your shift. Whether it's dealing with patient medication, dressing a wound, hanging an IV or calming a distressed patient, there is so much to do and seemingly not enough time to do it all. You can spend your time reacting to crises, ending up exhausted by the end of each shift.

Whether working in a bustling emergency department, a nursing home, a physician's clinic, or providing home healthcare, most likely you are frequently understaffed and overwhelmed, feeling the pressure to rush to get everything finished by the end of your shift.

Faced with constant pressure, with an endless list of tasks and chores, your mind may click into overdrive almost immediately. In such a state, you are less efficient at meeting the necessary tasks of the day. Like Stephanie, you might jump from task to task, dealing mindlessly with interruptions and emergencies as they arise.

Everything is of great importance, but not being able to set priorities and focus clearly on one task at a time can leave one feeling frazzled. In this mode, you may feel good about "getting things done." One by one, you cross off the "to-dos" from your list. As long as you are busy, you are being productive, right? Unfortunately, that's not always the case. And if you haven't taken the time to prioritize your tasks, you could miss doing something important simply because it was not next on the list.

When you attend to a task, or interact with a patient in a mindless way, you are not fully engaged with that experience. Even though you're physically present and you manage to do what needs to be done, your mind may be elsewhere.

Although this can obviously have negative consequences, it may not have serious health or safety implications. However, if you're not fully present for important nursing tasks such as inserting IVs', using overhead mechanical lifts, or preparing medications, the results can be very serious indeed. Have you ever injured yourself or someone else because you were just not thinking?

If you're not giving your undivided attention when administering medication, you may not realize that you are giving a medication that is inappropriate for the patient because the two names sound alike. Similarly, if your mind is elsewhere when you're using mechanical lifts, you may fail to properly secure the patient in the sling mechanism, causing a fall. Your failure to mindfully find the insertion point for your patient's IV can lead to more punctures and more pain for your patient.

Although you may not realize it at the time, these mindless work practices can endanger your patient and cause errors that have catastrophic consequences. In a busy environment where there is a lot to get done, it seems to make sense to juggle several tasks at once. Unfortunately, this can make things worse rather than better. When you are distracted or multi-tasking, your ability to take in or retain information can be impaired.

Instead of focusing clearly on doing one job at a time, you can end up doing several jobs inattentively. It is almost inevitable that sooner or later you will make a mistake. In nursing, this can be downright dangerous, and you can put lives at risk as well as jeopardize your own career.

If a doctor gives you orders for a patient and you forget what they are, you run the risk of making a life-threatening mistake. If you realize your error, you can contact the doctor for clarification but you will waste valuable time and may appear disorganized and unprofessional. Regardless of the outcome, chances are you will feel stressed and anxious, rather than calm and confident.

There is ample research available today that proves our brains cannot efficiently do many things at once. Instead, we use up a tremendous amount of brain energy switching between tasks. It actually takes more energy to multi-task than to do one thing at a time. No wonder being "productive" is so exhausting. Our brains weren't designed to switch between one task and another for extended periods of time.

In fact, people who multitask regularly are often unable to focus on what is important in life, compared with people who only multitask occasionally. So what's a frazzled, over-worked, and exhausted nurse supposed to do?

Fortunately, there is hope. Mindfulness practices can help to sharpen your attention, making it easier for you to notice danger or assess risk, both for your patients and yourself. As you move from patient to patient and task to task, you will be more vigilant and aware of potential hazards within your work environment. You may also notice the strain and stress that you put on your own mind and body.

With a mindful approach, you are able to work in a calmer, more intentional way, pay attention, prioritize tasks, and know when to shift gears and allow a task in progress to wait while you attend to another.

Mindfulness also helps you concentrate on tasks for longer, making you less prone to distractions and more able to quickly re-focus after being interrupted. Better concentration improves memory, boosts productivity, and reduces the stress involved in a busy workday. As you learn to focus on what you are doing and to cope better with distraction, you can be much more efficient and calm.

In short, mindfulness is an essential skill that every nurse should learn, and is, arguably, more important than many antiquated skills taught today such as mitering bed sheets and proper bed-bath techniques.

When you are present in this moment, you break the continuity of your story, of past and future. Then true intelligence arises, and also love.

—Eckhart Tolle

Mindfulness Defined

The ability to be fully present and attentive in the moment is one definition of mindfulness.

Indeed, many spiritual traditions emphasize this value of presence. Buddhism is the religion most often associated with mindfulness. For more than two thousand five hundred years, Buddhism has explored how mindfulness stills the mind and cultivates compassion. Anyone, however, can effectively practice mindfulness. You don't have to be Buddhist or follow any spiritual tradition.

Jon Kabat-Zinn, founder of Mindfulness-Based Stress Reduction (MBSR), defines mindfulness as "the awareness that arises from paying attention in a particular way: on purpose, in the present moment, and nonjudgmentally."[2] It is the practice of paying attention to what is going on both externally and internally in terms of thoughts, emotions, and sensations.

With the practice of mindfulness, you set your intention to pay attention:

- *On purpose,* by consciously and deliberately directing attention to your experience in the moment, be it a body sensation, a breath, an emotion, an interaction, or an activity. This purposeful and intentional direction of attention is a vital part of mindfulness.
- *In the present moment,* engaging with what is unfolding in the present, accepting it as it is, rather than getting caught up in habitual thoughts about the past and future.
- *Nonjudgmentally,* accepting whatever comes, whether it is sense perceptions, thoughts, or emotions, acknowledging them as they are, without labelling them as bad or good, pleasant or unpleasant, or judging them in any way.

Although this definition may sound uncomplicated, in reality, being present isn't always easy, especially in the environment of chronic stress that you may be exposed to daily. It is cultivated by being aware of what we are doing, thinking, and experiencing in the moment— accepting it without judgment — and then responding to it purposefully.

Like love, mindfulness is something that can't be fully understood until it is experienced and practiced. Think back to a moment in your life when you felt fulfilled, a moment that you still value and appreciate. What stands out most in your memory about this experience? Perhaps you were absorbed in a game with your

30

child, feeling a sense of awe when gazing at a breathtaking sunset, or experiencing the excitement of a new adventure. Maybe it was simply a look you shared with a special someone, or the smile of a stranger that touched your heart.

Can you remember what you were thinking back then, in that moment? Were you worrying about the past or obsessing about the future? Probably not. It was a moment of value precisely because you were really there for it, making it easy to recall and savor even now, possibly many years later. Moments like these are moments of mindfulness.

At the time, you might not have known the word or been familiar with the concept, but you were experiencing it just the same, through being fully present, and connecting with your experience. When you're mindful, you might notice the movement of breath in your body, the sensation of holding someone's hands, or how cool or warm the weather is. You might notice how you move your body when walking, the special way your loved one looks at you, and even the sounds of the leaves and the branches as they sway in the breeze.

Mindfulness is about being present in your life, with a clear awareness of what is happening, and being with your experience in a kind, open, and non-judging way. It has a quality of richness, where heart and mind are fully engaged, and where full attention is brought to the experience. Many people go through life in a perpetual state of *mindlessness*, functioning on autopilot with little awareness of the present moment.

How Mindful Are You?

Are you able to appreciate everyday life, or do you fall into the grip of daily stressors? Put simply, how mindful are you? In just ten minutes or less, you can get a sense of how mindful you are by rating yourself on the Mindful Attention Awareness Scale (MAAS):

Rate your Level of Mindfulness

Review the collection of statements [3] below in terms of your everyday experience. Using a one-to-six scale, indicate how frequently or infrequently you currently have each experience. Try to answer according to what really reflects your experience rather than what you think your experience should be. Consider each item separately from every other item.

Please Indicate the degree to which you agree with each of the following items using the scale below.		Almost always	Very frequently	Somewhat frequently	Somewhat Infrequently	Very Infrequently	Almost never
MAAS 1	I could be experiencing some emotion and not be conscious of it until sometime later.	□ 1	□ 2	□ 3	□ 4	□ 5	□ 6
MAAS 2	I break or spill things because of carelessness, not paying attention or thinking of something else.	□ 1	□ 2	□ 3	□ 4	□ 5	□ 6
MAAS 3	I find it difficult to stay focused on what's happening in the present	□ 1	□ 2	□ 3	□ 4	□ 5	□ 6
MAAS 4	I tend to walk quickly to get where I'm going without paying attention to what I experience along the way.	□ 1	□ 2	□ 3	□ 4	□ 5	□ 6
MAAS 5	I tend not to notice feelings of physical tension or discomfort until they really grab my attention.	□ 1	□ 2	□ 3	□ 4	□ 5	□ 6
MAAS 6	I forget a person's name almost as soon as I've been told It for the first time.	□ 1	□ 2	□ 3	□ 4	□ 5	□ 6
MAAS 7	It seems I am "running on automatic" without much awareness of what I'm doing.	□ 1	□ 2	□ 3	□ 4	□ 5	□ 6
MAAS 8	I rush through activities without being really attentive to them.	□ 1	□ 2	□ 3	□ 4	□ 5	□ 6
MAAS 9	I get so focused on the goal I want to achieve that I lose touch with what I am doing right now to get there.	□ 1	□ 2	□ 3	□ 4	□ 5	□ 6
MAAS 10	I do jobs or tasks automatically, without being aware of what I'm doing.	□ 1	□ 2	□ 3	□ 4	□ 5	□ 6
MAAS 11	I find myself listening to someone with one ear, doing something else at the same time.	□ 1	□ 2	□ 3	□ 4	□ 5	□ 6
MAAS 12	I drive places on automatic pilot and then wonder why I went there.	□ 1	□ 2	□ 3	□ 4	□ 5	□ 6
MAAS 13	I find myself preoccupied with the future or the past.	□ 1	□ 2	□ 3	□ 4	□ 5	□ 6
MAAS 14	I find myself doing things without paying attention.	□ 1	□ 2	□ 3	□ 4	□ 5	□ 6
MAAS 15	I snack without being aware that I'm eating	□ 1	□ 2	□ 3	□ 4	□ 5	□ 6

This version of the MAAS was reformatted by the Psychology Department, Ohio State University.

To score the questionnaire, simply compute a mean (average) of the fifteen items (add the scores and then divide by fifteen). Higher scores reflect higher levels of mindfulness. Typically, the average score is around 3.86. The highest score is 6, and the lowest score is 1.

Journal Reflection:

After scoring the scale, take a moment to reflect. Is your score what you expected? Did anything surprise you? Of the fifteen items, are any particularly relevant to your functioning as a nurse? If so, what are they and what are their implications? For example, items two, eight, and ten could have implications for safe practice. Similarly, items three, six, and eleven may reflect your ability to provide the support and teaching that are crucial to nursing practice. What kind of improvement do you hope to experience as you work through the practices in this book? You can take the questionnaire again when you reach the end of the book, to see how far you have come.

Mindful Moments

Although you may not always take the time to practice mindfulness consciously, nearly everyone has the ability to be mindful. Think of moments in your life where you were fully present, completely absorbed in what you were doing.

Have you ever been involved when a patient is coding? You and your colleagues are working as a well-oiled team. Your adrenaline is pumping, and you focus completely on the patient; you're thinking of nothing else. While you work the code, your attention is absorbed by saving that life.

Now think about other moments at work when you experienced this same kind of focused attention. Perhaps you comforted a frightened child in the emergency room when they required stitches, or a dying patient who had no family to rely on. How present did you feel? Mindfulness provides you with the key to switching on this focus at will, so that you can intentionally tune in to, and accept, your sensory experience as it unfolds in the present moment.

Consider This:

When assessing a patient, do you pay close attention to their breath sounds? Do you listen carefully to their apical heartbeat or just quickly check a peripheral pulse?

Do you rush through the assessment, hurrying to get to your next task?

Mindfulness helps you to be fully present during routine procedures and pay close attention to what you are doing. As you practice paying attention like this, you will likely find that the quality of your work improves. Importantly, when you are mindful in your nursing role, you are able to "see" your patients in their entirety, consider their physical condition and any abnormalities, listen to their complaints and tone of voice, observe their behavior and sense their mood, all of which contribute to a thorough nursing assessment and to building a plan of care. Most importantly, mindfulness helps you cultivate a different relationship with situations you find challenging or stressful.

Consider this example. Imagine you are walking into the operating room for your first day as a certified registered nurse anaesthetist. Thoughts flutter inside you like wind-driven clouds. They are scary thoughts. Will I be able to get the patient fully anesthetized? You may have images of the patient waking up during surgery or the surgeon becoming annoyed with your incompetence.

What if you fail to keep the patient's vital signs within normal limits during surgery? Will you be able to revive the patient after the surgery? Embarrassment and anxiety build inside you. Along with those emotions comes a pounding heart, shaking hands, and dry mouth, all combining to create a sense of dread, making you feel like you are going before a firing squad. The thoughts and images escalate to the point where you become so caught up in the drama that you have transformed a situation that is difficult, but manageable, into one that is frightening. This is typical of how you might stress yourself out when you are mindless. Perhaps you can relate to this scenario?

Imagine the very same scenario, but this time, you're being mindful. You walk into the operating room, aware of the impact the anticipation of what lies ahead is having on you. This awareness is the first step in doing things differently. Rather than being plunged into reactivity, you notice how your body, thoughts, and emotions are interacting to generate a fearful response. You're aware of the reactivity rising up inside you: the spinning thoughts, difficult emotions, and intense bodily sensations—the shallow breathing, palpitations, sweating. Once you can separate out the reality of what's happening from your *reaction* to it, chances are you will prevent yourself from being plunged into reactivity and be able to respond calmly to the situation instead.

When you check in with your thoughts, you see the narrative unfolding about how it's all going to go wrong, how you will fail, how your patient will suffer and you will feel humiliated. Once you become aware of the story you are telling yourself, you are no longer lost in the situation. You realize that the thoughts are simply things you are telling yourself about what might happen. The threat is imagined, not necessarily real. Being aware of your thoughts and acknowledging them helps you be less reactive in the face of this uncertain situation. This awareness allows you to step back from your thoughts. Once you are less identified with the narrative, the shallow breathing, palpitations, and sweating are more likely to subside, and you will feel less frazzled.

Mindfulness helps you to regulate your emotions so you can see the situation, including the tasks before you, more clearly. You take a breath and feel your feet on the floor, coming fully into your body. You remember you are part of a team, and a feeling of safety returns. In that moment, you are present, no longer lost in the scene as before, and things don't spiral downwards. You are able to pay careful attention to setting up of the IV, medications, and breathing equipment. Although you're aware there may be challenges in the process of surgery, you trust that you can handle them. Mindfulness has given you energy and clarity.

Mindfulness and Compassion-Based Research

For the past five years, mindfulness has begun revolutionizing the healthcare world. Literally hundreds of clinical studies show the powerful effect of MBSR interventions. For healthcare workers, mindfulness interventions consistently and demonstrably reduce their stress, improve their self-compassion, and increase the effectiveness of their patient care.

As you work through this book, you will be able to try for yourself the various MBSR practices that research has shown to be effective in reducing the types of stress, burnout, and anxiety that affect everyone, including nurses like you, as well as other healthcare professionals.[4]

You will find that these simple practices, many of which take only moments to do and can be done anywhere, also improve your compassion, empathy, focus, and mood. Practitioners often report that they feel better about themselves and their work. Neuroscience backs up these subjective findings. In fact, scientists who scanned the brains of people practicing mindfulness found that physical changes occur in the brain's structure when people incorporate mindfulness into their lives. The scientists documented how the parts of the brain associated with memory, empathy, self-regulation, and executive control strengthen with mindfulness practice.[5] Mindfulness is not just a "feel-good" practice, but one that also has demonstrable benefits, as supported by scientific research.

Like mindfulness, compassion is triggering a scientific revolution, with research showing how compassion practice also changes the brain. Compassion is deeply rooted in our brains and bodies, so it has a biological basis. Dr. Dacher Keltner, a research psychologist at the University of California, Berkeley, wrote that our brains are wired to respond to the suffering of others: "We're wired to care. If you feel pain, a part of your brain lights up, and if you see someone have physical pain, that same part of your brain lights up."[6]

Not only are we wired to care for others, but remarkably, we also get the same pleasure from helping others as we get from gratifying our own personal desires. They say that virtue is its own reward. Well, being a compassionate person who does kind things also brings its own rewards. We feel better about ourselves, about our lives, and our world. But that's not the only benefit. Our health and longevity also improve.

Moreover, when you feel compassion, your heart rate slows, and you release oxytocin, the hormone that promotes bonding behavior. A warm smile, genuine hug, or friendly body language is enough to release this hormone in your body. When you feel caring toward others, it has a ripple effect, generating a chemical reaction in your body that leads to even more compassionate behavior.

Resilience to stress increases with compassion as you become more able to manage the feelings provoked by another person's distress and to feel concerned and motivated to help. Indeed, programs with a "loving-kindness" component have generated the best results for healthcare practitioners.[7] Later in this book, you will learn how to cultivate loving-kindness, by extending goodwill and kindheartedness to yourself and others.

Journal Reflection:

What is your intention in reading this book?

What are you hoping for?

In what ways do you feel mindfulness and compassion practice might change the way you live and work?

Moving toward Mindfulness: Two Forms of Practice

Mindfulness practice comes in two distinct forms: formal and informal. Formal practices include sitting meditation, mindful movement, walking meditation, and body scans (which you will learn in Chapter 6). These practices require setting aside a certain time in the day to deliberately practice presence and cultivate awareness. Informal practice, on the other hand, includes being mindful during everyday activities and interactions, and can be done anytime, anywhere. Both formal and informal practices are of equal importance. Each nourishes the other, and together both will nourish your life and your nursing practice.

Mindfulness of Breathing

There is possibly no better way to return to the present than deliberately bringing attention to your breathing, which is the most fundamental thing we all do to stay alive. What makes breathing so useful as a focus for returning to the present is that we can connect with the act of breathing at any moment. Since breathing is always available to us, we can access it at any time to become present and restore balance and stability.

Mindful breathing is a sitting meditation that involves bringing attention back to the breath, again and again, when it wanders. It is a process of sensing the breath, and attending to it, with a kind, nonjudgmental attention. Regular practice helps train your attention and tame the monkey mind.

To meditate with mindful breathing is to bring body and mind back to the present moment so that you do not miss your appointment with life.

—Thich Nhat Hanh

Most of the time, breathing happens outside of awareness; you don't notice it. When practicing mindful breathing, you ground yourself in the present moment by focusing on the breath. (To access a guided audio recording of mindful breathing, visit www.nursingmindfully.com.)

Try This:
Mindful Breathing

Set your timer for five minutes.

Sit in a comfortable chair, allowing the eyes to close gently.

Gradually become aware of the sensations of breathing wherever you feel them most. Perhaps you feel the breath passing through the nostrils or maybe your focus is on the rhythmic movements of the chest or abdomen.

Notice each breath as it unfolds, letting your attention settle there.

Not long after you begin focusing on the breath, your monkey mind will start acting up with a torrent of thoughts: "I wonder how long I've been doing this…When I finish, I'm going to have a coffee…I can't imagine how this can possibly help me."

The first thought will rapidly snare onto the next thought, and before you know it, the thoughts will snowball, sweeping you away with them in a storyline—blaming, stressing, or planning.

This is not a problem. It's simply what the mind does. When you notice your attention has wandered off into thoughts, you can simply mentally say to yourself: "thinking."

Then, gently and kindly bring your attention back to your breath, not judging it for wandering, but accepting that this is what the mind does naturally. This will help to calm that monkey!

No matter how many times your attention wanders, patiently bring it back to your breath. Remember, your breath is your anchor, bringing you back to the here and now.

To end this practice, gradually widen your awareness to the space around you, slowly opening your eyes and bringing your attention back into the room again.

Journal Reflection:

Take a moment to reflect on your experience of doing this practice for the first time.

What did you notice?

What difficulties did you have in focusing on the breath?

How are you feeling right now?

Busy Shifts

Here is an example of how mindful breathing can help you cope during a busy shift. Your shift starts like any other, full force, with constant, distracting background noise: patients, nurses and doctors conversing, the clattering of medical equipment, a ringing telephone, and footsteps running back and forth. You also carry your own distractions: a rush of inner thoughts and a buzzing cell phone. No doubt, these all take a toll on your focus.

When you enter your patient's room, you realize that you forgot to bring his medications. Feeling embarrassed and stressed, you return to the medication room. The truth is this might happen a lot more frequently than you care to admit. Days like this can contribute to burnout and nurse turnover.

By contrast, if you spend a few minutes at the beginning of your shift practicing mindful breathing, you will start your shift feeling more grounded and focused. Afterwards, you can more easily focus, list your priorities, and decide what you most need to accomplish to stay on task. You stock your scrub pockets with supplies so that you can avoid unnecessary trips to pick up alcohol wipes or tape. Also, your personal phone is turned off to ensure it will not interrupt your interactions with staff and patients.

Now that you have a clear sense of your tasks and have the tools to accomplish them, your attention can focus on the immediate needs of your patients. If you begin your shift with calm attention and a clear set of priorities, everything will run more smoothly. And if you tune in to your breathing throughout the day, you will be able to stay steady and calm, as Tanya Roberts, an ER nurse, describes: "Mindful breathing works for me when I'm in the midst of a particularly busy day, with a never-ending list of things to do. Rather than getting inundated with thoughts about what needs to be done next and how I'm never going to find the time to do it all, I let my breath calm and steady me. Stepping back from thoughts gives me space and helps me pause. Not only do I feel calmer, but I actually get more done!"

Practice Every Day

To plant the seed of mindfulness firmly in your life, set the intention to practice mindful breathing daily. You might think to yourself, "I don't have time to do this every day." Remember, you don't have to meditate for long stretches at a time. In fact, you can start off very simply with as little as five minutes a day, gradually increasing the time. Mindful breathing gives you a strong support for the rest of your practice, making it much easier to be mindful during the rest of the day.

At first, as with developing any new habit, it will likely be challenging, but it is a habit worth cultivating, as the benefits will ripple out beyond the formal sitting to all the activities you engage in throughout your day.

Nurse Mary Wilbur has observed how nurses work harder nowadays and with fewer resources. She suggests that the busy nurse can expand the day by spending thirty minutes or less in meditation. She notes that mindfulness practices are not radical, cost nothing, are simple to do, and enable nurses to focus on what's important and avoid getting distracted. Highlighting how meditation improved her life, Nurse Wilbur writes: "My desk is clear. My work is caught up. I don't feel the frustrations as keenly as before."[8] Most nurses can easily relate to the desire and the need to be more focused in daily life. Do you need more convincing?

Informal Practice: Daily Mindfulness

Meditation is a microcosm, a model, a mirror. The skills we practice when we sit are transferable to the rest of our lives.

—Sharon Salzberg

When you practice mindfulness in a formal way, like the sitting meditation you just did, in time you will experience the benefits Nurse Wilbur described. And the practice doesn't have to end the moment you get up and continue with your day. Rather, you can practice informally by taking this honed attention into your daily activities and any challenges you encounter.

Informal mindfulness is about bringing full awareness to the rest of your life, living your life fully and mindfully. At your disposal any moment of your day, it is a mobile practice, requiring no props or equipment, and it's free. Any routine activity can become a mindfulness practice when you give it your full attention.

It works like this: remind yourself to pay attention to and accept the reality of what is occuring in the moment, whether you're on the phone, doing rounds, charting, interacting with a difficult patient, or hanging an IV. Just as with mindful sitting, you guide your attention back to the point of focus—in this case, the task at hand—when you notice attention has wandered. By becoming more aware and present to what is happening in each moment of your day, you can begin to untangle yourself from difficult emotions and mental preoccupations. Then you are more able to regulate how you feel and will be less likely to get caught up in playing out old, automatic, and unhelpful, patterns of living and thinking.

Practicing informally helps you to get the full benefit from formal practice and integrate mindfulness into your everyday life. Just as formal practice becomes part of your daily routine, eventually cultivating the ability to be mindful throughout the day will also come naturally, and you will find that life is a lot less stressful.

Everything is grist for the mindfulness mill. Conflicts with coworkers, less-than-sympathetic supervisors, and patients who become very sick very quickly can be challenges that you now choose to meet with mindfulness and compassion.

In the next chapter, we will explore how to increase mindfulness by identifying the difference between *being* and *doing* in your everyday life.

Practice Plan:

Practice mindful breathing for five minutes daily. Tune in to the breath at intervals throughout your day, and notice any effects that mindful breathing has on your mind, body, and emotions. Reflect on your experience in your journal.

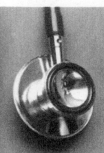
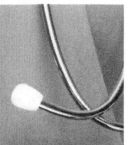

Points to Remember

✦ Mindfulness teaches you how to pay attention on purpose, in the present moment, without judgment.

✦ Just like mindfulness, compassion has been shown to benefit psychological health, resilience, and overall well-being.

✦ Mindfulness is not a quick fix; maintain realistic expectations.

✦ You can practice mindfulness formally as well as informally in your everyday activities.

✦ By becoming mindful and compassionate, you learn to be less reactive in stressful situations.

CHAPTER TWO

Doing and Being

It takes great courage and energy to cultivate non-doing,
both in stillness and in activity.

—Jon Kabat-Zinn

Do you ever feel panic at the end of a long weekend or vacation, wondering where the time went? Do your days, weeks, and months blend into one another, each day bringing you more of the same?

The profession of nursing has moved from task orientation to critical thinking, which has increased the complexity of the work and the opportunity for errors. At work, you move through a series of tasks so that patient care runs smoothly—you assess your patients, change drips, review test results. However, you may be on autopilot the entire time, lost in *doing* and unaware of the present in which you are *being*.

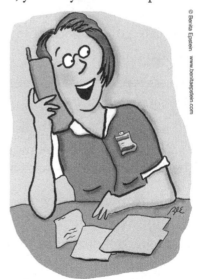

Betty worked on a busy cancer treatment floor for about two years. She was a go-getter, volunteering for projects that she didn't need to do. In fact, she loved nursing because she had the satisfaction of helping others and solving complex problems. As Betty methodically worked through her to-do list during her shift, she resented being interrupted to address anything that was not on her schedule.

"Oh, me? Nothing much. I treated a dozen patients, did the charts, wrote new protocols, gave a seminar, fixed the computer and now it's lunchtime."

45

Betty would whizz from room to room, getting the job done but not focusing on much else. Obsessed by her list of tasks, she did not take time to talk to patients or coworkers. In the end, she was so consumed with getting her tasks done and checking off the boxes on her list that she forgot what it meant to connect with her patients. Yet, Betty couldn't help noticing that her patient's eyes lit up when her colleague entered the room. She envied the rapport this colleague had with his patients and began to realize that she was missing out.

Betty needed to change the way she approached her work. Instead of obsessing over her list, she needed to let go and start being more present for herself, her patients, and her coworkers.

Perhaps, like Betty, you have spent entire shifts in *doing* mode and missed out on connecting with yourself and your patients? That's not to say that *doing* is a bad place to be. On the contrary, *doing* mode is an important part of everyday life—it helps you plan your day, finish the tasks you started, and pay attention to detail. In the same way, *doing* mode helps you manage your daily routine from driving in traffic to shopping for dinner to paying bills. But once you complete your tasks, it is important to switch out of *doing* mode and simply *be* in the moment.

DOING Mode: Goal-oriented, focused on getting things done, restless, conceptual

BEING Mode: In the moment, aware, allowing, accepting

Think of it this way: *doing* would be your mode if you were planning a romantic anniversary dinner. You would choose the restaurant, get directions, and drive there. Once you arrived, though, you would want to enjoy your meal and the time with your loved one. That is when you would switch to *being* mode. Obviously, it is important to be able to switch off *doing* mode after its job is done and enjoy life. Imagine if you were to spend your romantic dinner checking traffic patterns for the drive home!

All nurses are familiar with *doing* mode. Your training emphasizes it, and in a profession that is task-driven, being busy is valued. Yet, when you are constantly in *doing* mode, your monkey mind leaps from one thought to the next, you forget about the moment you're in, and after a while, your feelings control you. Unable to switch out of *doing* mode, and hijacked by whatever thought or emotion pops up, you end up merely going through the motions, just like Betty.

Operating this way makes you lose touch with what is going on right there in the moment. For example, if your mind is on other things when you drink your coffee, you don't really taste it. If you spend your break reviewing lab results, you've not enjoyed *your* moment in the present to re-group and re-charge. What details are you missing when you are always *doing*? How about the smiles and hellos from visitors and colleagues, the beautiful flower arrangement at the nurses' station, the great sunrise out the window, or the opportunity to say "thanks" to the person who opens the door?

If you're stuck in *doing* mode when you meet your first patient, you miss the opportunity to make a real connection. The present sails past and never comes back. That moment is lost forever.

Autopilot

In your eagerness to get things done, you can become so absorbed in your thoughts that you don't notice what is going on inside or around you. Have you ever missed your stop on the bus because you were daydreaming? Or put your keys in the fridge while talking on the phone? Have you ever entered the medication room and stared at the shelves, unable to remember what you went in there for or what you needed? Or maybe you started up your computer to check a lab value but couldn't remember what value you were looking for or why.

Rather than focusing on the task at hand, you are on "autopilot," absentmindedly going through the motions. If you're "autopiloting" a lot, sooner or later, you will trip up and make mistakes.

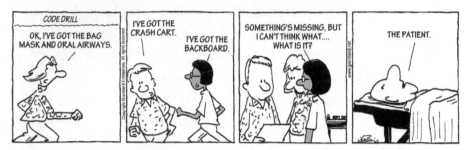

On autopilot, you focus on the result rather than giving full attention to the task at hand. That said, autopilot is not always a bad thing. In fact, it's important. The brain's ability to switch into this mode allows you to complete complex tasks like driving or using a computer without thinking about all the detailed actions involved. Thus, being on autopilot allows you to avoid expending unnecessary energy on routine things. However, sometimes you forget to come out of autopilot and fixate instead on the next urgent task on your to-do list. Research has shown that the average person spends 47% of the time on autopilot.[9] Rather than having a sense of really living, if you're trapped on constant autopilot, you will likely feel exhausted and dissatisfied with life. Remember to take an occasional break from *doing* to help you connect with yourself and others and recharge your batteries.

Mindful Presence

Being present is infinitely more powerful than anything you can say or do.
—Eckhart Tolle

In the course of your workday, you may be on autopilot while you're with your patient, preoccupied by your never-ending workload and urgent to-do lists. Although your time together may be limited, how can you spend the precious time you *do* have together in a heartful way where your patient feels your caring presence?

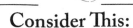

Consider This:

Imagine that you're in conversation with a patient. You're completely present during the interaction. The patient feels a genuine connection with you. Because you have been mindful during the conversation, the person feels you are really listening. They trust what you say. They feel comfortable, content, and at ease in your presence. Can you sense how mindful presence can enrich your work as a nurse?

Try This:
Mindful Presence

Before you enter a patient's room, scan your body for sensations. Perhaps your jaw is clenched or your shoulders are tense.

Notice any sense of feeling rushed or anxious, and acknowledge these feelings without trying to get rid of them.

Take some mindful breaths, letting your tension and busyness dissolve on the exhale.

As you get ready to meet your patient, set the intention to be fully present.

Knock on the door and establish eye contact as you enter the patient's room.

Introduce yourself warmly and make a connection.

Chat together for a moment or two before moving on to the assessment or placing your fingers on the computer keyboard.

Whenever you notice your attention has wandered, gently bring it back to your patient and the task at hand.

Set the intention to give your patient your full attention during each interaction. Unhook from the busyness of your day, come off autopilot, and take a moment to become grounded.

Mindful presence doesn't take more time. Instead, it adds value—it makes every moment count.

Balancing Doing and Being

For most of us, a typical day involves hurrying from task to task, forgetting that there are other possibilities for us. Even a tiny bit of mindfulness, brought to any moment, can wake us up, thus subverting the momentum of doing for at least one moment.

—*The Mindful Way through Depression*, by Mark Williams, John Teasdale, Zindel Segal, and Jon Kabat-Zinn

Throughout the day, you continually oscillate between *doing* and *being* modes. When you are in *doing* or autopilot mode, you might spike and hang an IV bag while talking to the patient and thinking of what you need to do in the next room. Obviously, this is a lot to focus on at once.

Doing is a mechanical, cerebral mode in which you can prioritize events, make lists, and focus on tasks. Although this mode is important to your function as a nurse, it may stop you from being fully present because you are preoccupied and lost in thought.

How do you see your personal balance, at work and in your personal life? Are you more often in *doing* than in *being* mode? To answer that question, consider the statements that follow. Which ones apply to you? If you recognize yourself in four or more of the following statements, then you are spending a lot of time in *doing* mode.

☐   On your way to the hospital or facility, you're concerned with reaching your destination or preparing your to-do list. You don't notice the fresh breeze coming in the car window or the family of birds flying overhead.

☐ It's difficult to focus on what's happening in the present. Perhaps you're completing your electronic medical record, but you're thinking of the new orders you've been given, the family with questions, and the return phone call to your child's teacher, all begging for your attention right now.

☐ You feel like you're constantly running on autopilot. Your everyday experiences come and go without much awareness. You don't notice the sensation of changing crisp white sheets, don't feel the reward of a patient's laughter, and miss out on the joking staff camaraderie.

☐ You rush through your tasks—whipping through assessments, medications, rounds, charting—always focused on the end result and what remains to be done.

☐ You don't stop to connect with your patient. Preoccupied, your hand poised on the doorknob, you only half-listen because your attention has moved on to the next task.

☐ You think a lot about the past and future, not paying attention to the present.

☐ You become easily stressed and frustrated.

☐ You don't notice physical tension or discomfort until you're in pain.

Journal Reflection:

How much of your day do you spend in *doing* mode?

Switching from *Doing* to *Being*

If you are spending too much time in *doing* mode, you're not alone, as this is common to most people. Fortunately, you do not need to be trapped in an endless cycle. You can change this by focusing on the present, not the past or future, and on the process, not the result. In the middle of all the hectic activity, you can be mindful and cultivate *being* mode. To do this, you can choose to be accepting, aware, and open to what is unfolding, rather than being lost in the rush and flow of thinking and *doing*.

Remember, you can still be busy and engaged in doing things when you tap into *being* mode. The difference is that, rather than being lost in thought, you are fully present and aware of what is happening within and around you. For instance, instead of rehashing the confrontation you had with a colleague earlier, you give your undivided attention to taking your patient's vital signs, right now. In doing so, your mind becomes less reactive and more concentrated, and your work benefits.

> *"Being" is what slows down the nurse so that space is created for an authentic, deep connection with the patient and healing. The work of "being" has remained constant over time. Embedded in the "being" dimension of the role lies the essence of nursing.*
>
> —Joellen Goertz Koerner

You are in *being* mode when you are fully present with the patient, the doctor, the family, or your loved one. You are not lost in judgments or jumping ahead in your mind to the next task demanding your attention. *Being* mode is just as essential as doing mode to nursing because it allows you to connect to your experience on a deeper level. In the end, it is the very essence of mindfulness.

Spending time in *being* mode allows you to experience your day in a completely new way. For example, when you're driving, you might be using *doing* mode to focus on reaching your destination. However, if you slip into *being* mode, then you are present for the experience of driving itself, feeling your body in the seat and your hands on the steering wheel, noticing any tension or stress, as well as appreciating the sights along your way. Taking time to *be* in this way may help silence the continual to-do list rattling around in your mind and, instead, you can enjoy relaxing.

At work, think about those special moments when you experience a deep connection with a patient, when you feel fully present as you listen, share, and connect. These are moments of *being*.

A good way to stop all the doing is to shift into the 'being mode' for a moment. [...] Just watch this moment, without trying to change it at all. What is happening? What do you feel? What do you see? What do you hear?

—Jon Kabat-Zinn

Everyday *Being*

At any time during your day, you can switch to *being* mode and free yourself from the constant stress of *doing*. Changing from *doing* to *being* takes practice and may seem elusive at first. Since the average nursing shift is fast-paced with a high workload, remembering to slow down and enter *being* mode can be challenging. You may start your shift feeling relaxed, but after an hour of rushing around, you're back in your habitual frenzied mode, with your mind racing and your body feeling overworked. Whether you're helping a patient to the bathroom or calling for housekeeping, you are lost in action, unaware of what is going on inside or around you. However, with regular practice, you start to notice what mode you're in during the day and can more easily switch to the mode required for the task at hand. Mindfulness will become a habit.

A simple way to get started is to assign the role of reminder to certain objects in your environment or to certain moments in your routine. These reminders then serve the function of bringing you back to the present when your attention inevitably wanders during the day. The reminder could be the sight of a patient's room number, a sign for contact precautions, or taking your favorite pen out of your pocket. You need only mentally assign some object or routine event with the role of "trigger," of reminding you to come back to the present. Then, whenever you encounter the trigger, you will automatically remember to be mindful in that moment.

The Family Medicine Program at the Wisconsin University School of Medicine[10] developed a simple practice called the 3 Ps, which is particularly suitable for nurses who are used to opening doors repeatedly in the course of a workday.[11] Let's try this out right now.

Try This:
The 3 Ps

As you open the door to a patient's room, use the doorknob as the trigger to practice the 3 Ps. When reaching for the door knob, take a moment to do the following:

Pause. Take a breath and let go of *doing* mode.

Be Present. Notice your bodily sensations, as well as your thoughts and emotions, accepting whatever is present.

Proceed. Respond skillfully to what needs attention, using mindful speech and action.

Journal Reflection:

After trying out the 3 Ps, take a moment to reflect on your experience.

What did you notice?

How did it feel to shift from *doing* to *being*?

Fortunately, you don't need to stop what you are doing to access *being* mode. As often as you remember to do so, explore *being* mode during activities at home or at work. Pause for a few moments before powering on the computer, picking up the handheld infrared scanner, or touching the keyboard. Focus your attention on the here and now. Feel your feet on the floor and take some mindful breaths.

Louise Conrad, a midwife, told me about her experience of using a mindfulness trigger. "As soon as my shift started, I would immediately click into overdrive and often feel frazzled. I decided to make one simple change. Whenever I passed through a doorway, I took a moment to connect with my breath. The doorway was my cue to notice if I was over-thinking, and to come back to the present. This simple moment of mindfulness was restorative. It gave me permission to come off overdrive and into the moment."

From *Doing* to *Being*

Being mode is always available, even in the midst of busyness, and you can move from *doing* to *being* in a moment. For example, you can be working intensely in the middle of a code and yet be conscious of the knot in your stomach, and the anxious thoughts and feelings that are present. Taking a few deep breaths and feeling your feet in contact with the ground will place you in the present and change your physiology from wired to calm.

Practice Plan:

This week, continue to practice mindful breathing for five to ten minutes daily.

Choose an object you encounter at work as a cue to practice the 3 Ps. Whenever you encounter this "trigger," pause for a moment, focus on your breathing, and bring your attention to what you are doing. Reflect on your experience in your journal.

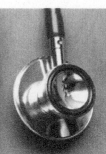
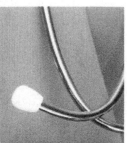

Points to Remember

+ You may be in *doing* mode much of the time and unaware of *being*.
+ In *doing* mode, you complete everyday tasks on autopilot.
+ On autopilot, you're disconnected from your senses and unaware of the present.
+ When you are in *being* mode, you're in the present rather than being lost in the past or future.
+ Spending time *being* has many benefits, including a greater sense of calm and self-awareness.
+ Mindfulness practice cultivates the ability to choose to enter *being* mode.

CHAPTER THREE

Everyday Mindfulness

Each place is the right place
—the place where I now am can be a sacred space.

—Ravi Ravindra

You may wonder how you can fit mindfulness into your daily schedule. At work, you put in grueling hours in an understaffed department, often working extra shifts. At home, chasing children, doing laundry, and catching up with housecleaning—not to mention trying to have a social life—all take up your precious off-hours. Divide your attention among all your responsibilities and suddenly you don't remember whether you ate lunch or who you talked with on the phone. Life happens in a blur.

Who has time to smell the proverbial roses, let alone to spend twenty or thirty minutes meditating?

Consider This:

Have you ever been introduced to someone only to forget their name thirty seconds later? Have you ever finished a lunch break but can't recall a half hour later what you ate? Have you ever taken a patient's vital signs, left the room to write them down, but forgotten your findings by the time you put pen to paper?

These "little forgetful moments" are all too common among nurses who juggle enormous workloads. Yet they can make your workload feel even heavier.

Don't worry. No matter how busy you are, the beauty of mindfulness is that there are many opportunities to practice it *informally* each day. You can be mindful even in the midst of routine work tasks, like measuring blood pressure or preparing a patient for surgery.

Mary Chris Coen is a nurse straight out of school and working her first professional nursing job on a cardiac step-down unit. Part of her orientation focused on using mindfulness for stress reduction. She took these practices to heart and used them to help slow down her racing mind and ease into the stressful world of nursing.

"The most important thing I learned was to remember to breathe," she says. "Even when I'm tired and extremely busy, when I remember to pause for a few seconds and take a mindful breath, it makes a world of difference. It brings me right back to the moment I'm in."

Most of the time, Mary Chris is running through her day with no space to take time out. Despite that, she manages to bring full attention to each activity during her shift. For example, as she prepares to administer medications, she remembers to focus on each patient, visualizing their face, their medical issues, and the reason for the medications. By completing each step the same way every time, she is being mindful of her responsibility to that patient and is fully engaged, reducing the risk of mistakes and providing herself a sense of accomplishment.

"Being mindful doesn't take more time," she says. "It just means that I stay present with what I'm doing right now."

Mary Chris impressed her preceptor and manager with her lack of medication errors, and she received high marks in her initial evaluation for her close attention to detail.

This chapter will show you how to intentionally focus, like Mary Chris, on being in the present, as you go about your daily tasks—even those you find frustrating or repetitive. By bringing mindfulness to your daily routine, you will feel less stressed and be more effective in your work. As a result, you may even discover a renewed appreciation for the work you do.

Starting Out

When you start practicing mindfulness, it can be difficult to let go of worries and frustrations. Have patience with yourself. No one is perfect, and your busy brain is bound to fight back at first. You might feel that your time would be better spent getting more done. If that's how you feel, try not to pressure yourself. Above all, don't think of mindfulness practice as yet another thing to add to your to-do list!

Start with the intention to do *just one* activity mindfully. For example, can you be fully present when brushing your teeth in the morning? What about while having dinner with your family… without a cell phone to answer staffing calls? Even if you can only be mindful for one minute of every day, congratulate yourself for that minute of mindfulness.

Mindful Driving

On a typical drive to work, your mind may be focused on the shift ahead, making a mental list of all the things that need doing. You think about the patients who need your attention and worry whether your sick coworker will be back today to share the load. Maybe you're planning a belated comeback to a rude colleague. Before you know it, you've arrived at work without noticing anything along the way.

It is little wonder, then, that the workday can feel like a struggle when you have spent the first part of your morning worrying about things outside of your control. Instead of stressing out on your commute, use the time to focus on what is happening right now. Start by driving a little more slowly, and noticing what's around you.

What is the weather like? Is there more traffic than usual? Pay close attention to any physical sensations, and be aware of the sounds of traffic, construction noise, or the music playing on your car radio. Remember to bring your attention to the feel of the air on your skin and the scents, pleasant or otherwise, that surround you.

Be aware of drivers approaching you from behind. Share the road rather than fight for territory; make an effort to drive calmly, braking and accelerating as smoothly as possible. See if you can come to a complete stop without jerking the car—no slamming on the brakes! When you encounter stop-and-go traffic or when other drivers cut you off, try not to judge the experience as "bad": let it be a reminder to breathe and be in the moment. Any time traffic slows, take a few moments to focus on your breathing. When you become distracted by thoughts such as work, family, or money, identify the distraction, let it go, and gently bring yourself back to the present. In short, enjoy this little window of time by yourself!

Imelda Gallagher, a cardiac nurse, began incorporating mindful driving into her journey to work. "As I sat in my car, I would focus on my breath, and relax any tension. When my mind would jump to thoughts about the day ahead, I would bring my attention right back to the present. It made such a difference. When I began my day with mindful driving, I started to feel less stressed at work. I was more relaxed and felt less overwhelmed."

If, like Imelda, you stay mindful during your morning commute, you will begin your shift feeling less stressed, and you can continue being mindful by "single tasking" like this throughout your day.

Arriving at Work

Once you arrive at your workplace, take a moment to self-assess. Do you notice any tightness in your muscles as you approach the building? Are you carrying any worries with you?

Take this opportunity to relax into *being* mode. For example, as you walk to the entrance, notice your breathing and gently focus on completing an inhale-exhale cycle. In the same way, pay attention to the act of walking, observing how you move each foot and place it on the ground.

Take a few moments to center yourself before entering the building. If worries about the demands of the day intrude, notice them and bring your awareness back to your breathing.

When you get to the nurses' station or your desk, notice whether you have slipped back into *doing* mode. Again, take a few breaths and return to your mindful way of being.

Mindful Eating

As you move through your day, rushing from patient to patient, preparing medications, keeping up with the steady stream of new orders, stress builds. When you finally have a moment or two to squeeze in lunch, you grab something quick from the cafeteria or vending machine and wolf it down. But at what cost to your own health and well-being? You put so much into the care of others, shouldn't your lunch be

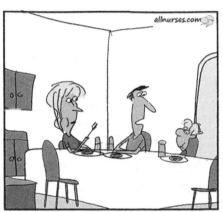

"Yes, your mom did finish her meal in 2 minutes. It's a habit a nurse picks up after being constantly bothered on her lunch hour."

as nourishing for you as lunch should be for your patients? Mindful eating improves digestion and reconnects you with the present.

There are some people who eat an orange but don't really eat it.
They eat their sorrow, fear, anger, past, and future.

—Thich Nhat Hanh

Try This:
Mindful Eating

To get started, choose a time when you have a moment to sit by yourself, and take a few cleansing breaths.

Now, look at your food, observing the various shapes and colors, feeling the weight of the food as you pick it up with your utensils. If it is something you eat with your hands, gently run your fingertips along its surface, feeling the texture and temperature and inhaling the scent.

Put the food in your mouth—but don't start chewing yet. Take your time. To avoid the thought of your next bite distracting you, put down the utensil or the food in your hand as you focus on eating one bite mindfully. How does it taste? Feel the texture on your tongue. Is it smooth or lumpy? Warm or cold? As you move the food around in your mouth, does it melt? Do you sense new flavors emerging?

Notice the movement in your mouth as you chew. Listen to the sound. Is it crunchy? Pay attention to the act of swallowing. Continue eating mindfully throughout your meal. Notice as your body begins to feel satisfied. How much food is left on your plate when your body feels full?

A nurse named Eileen Cameron who works in a pediatric orthopedic surgeon's office told how sitting down to a leisurely meal was a rarity for her. "Being a busy nurse, I regularly skipped meals and always grabbed breakfast on the run. Food was simply fuel for my body. Mindful eating has helped me to really taste my food, and also to notice how certain foods make me feel energized or bloated and tired. Now, I make better choices and eat the kind of food that supports me to do my work. I listen to my body and intuitively know what it needs. And I make a point of starting each day with a mindful breakfast."

Mindful eating is a big challenge for most busy people, but especially for nurses who are accustomed to quick meals while on duty! Yet, like Eileen, you can practice mindful eating at every opportunity. Focus on slowing down, and savoring your food, if only for a few moments. When you practice eating mindfully, you may become more selective when choosing your food because you will know what gives you energy, what helps you feel nourished, and which tastes are pleasant enough to repeat!

For more guidance on beginning the journey of mindful eating, read Thich Nhat Hanh and Lillian Cheung's book *Savor: Mindful Eating, Mindful Life*. This book is a great resource.

Journal Reflection:

After you practice mindful eating, take a moment to reflect on your experience. How did it feel different from the way you normally eat?

Anchor Activity

When you're in the throes of a hectic shift juggling multiple tasks, mindfulness may feel like a luxury you cannot afford. However, that's the time you need it most!

To get going, decide on an activity to anchor you in the course of your workday. You can choose any task as your *anchor activity*, to bring you out of autopilot and into the present. While doing that task, become aware of your breathing and of what is going on inside and around you.

A good example of a possible anchor activity is hand washing. As a nurse, you wash your hands many times a day, and you can use this ritual as an opportunity to come back into connection with yourself. This way, you can turn a routine task into a moment of presence, one that you can repeat as the hours go by.

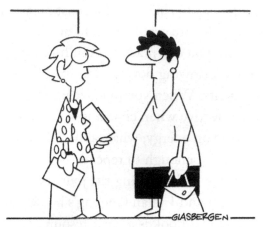

"Nurses work 12 hours a day: 4 hours caring
for patients and 8 hours washing our hands."

Try This:
Mindful Handwashing

Step out of your monkey mind and soap up your hands as though you were doing it for the very first time. Slow down and be deliberate in your actions. Feel each sensation: the warm water on your skin and the smell of the soap. Take time to wash each finger, the backs of your hands, between your fingers, and up to your wrists.

Feel your feet anchored to the floor and the weight of your hands as they move over each other.

Become aware of any sense of aliveness and vitality in your hands, noticing the simple pleasure of warm water on your skin and enjoying the feeling of clean hands.

Picture all stress and worry spiraling down the drain with the water. As you dry your hands, continue being mindfully present, noticing all the sensations. No matter how many times you wash and dry your hands, each moment is refreshingly unique.

Although this might seem like an extravagant amount of time, especially in the current day of hand-sanitizer short-cuts, not only are you being present and mindful of the task, you are choosing *not* to take shortcuts. In the end, you may find that hospital acquired infections (HAI) or nosocomial infections actually decrease on your unit. Now, that's a systemic change from which everyone can benefit!

Emily Quinn, a nurse in ICU, has found this practice so useful: "For me, washing my hands was always something I did quickly and mechanically, so that I could get it over and done with and move on to my next task. Lately, I've come to realize this simple activity is actually a powerful mindfulness practice and one that I can use again and again during a busy shift. Afterwards, I move on to my next clinical duty, feeling centered and energized."

Be Mindful of Your Senses

Whenever you notice that your mind is distracted as you move through your day, use any one of your five senses to come back to the present. Often you may be so lost in thought that you have little awareness of the sensations of touching, tasting, smelling, hearing, and seeing. Yet it is these sensations that bring you into the here and now. It is also these senses that nurses have honed throughout their career. They make up your "gut feeling" and your "intuition." They tell you when something is wrong and how to move forward.

When you notice that you're lost in action and your mind is spinning, bring your attention to any one of your senses. Scan your environment, really taking in your surroundings. What can you see, hear, touch, taste, or smell?

Can you feel your stethoscope around your neck or the weight of your pen and supplies in your pockets? Do you notice the light coming in through the window or reflecting off the monitors? Can you feel the air circulating or still against your skin?

You can draw on this simple practice many times throughout your day to unhook from thinking and ground yourself in the present moment.

Use every opportunity to practice throughout your day. For instance, as you assess each patient, take time to notice the sound of each breath. Listen closely for crackles, rales, and even diminished breath sounds. If you notice the impulse to move on quickly to assessing heart sounds, gently bring yourself back to the moment, noticing the coolness of the stethoscope in your hand and the sensations of the buds in your ears. Take a moment to connect with your breath and notice any feelings, whether pleasant or unpleasant.

Foundational Attitudes

Practicing mindfulness, no matter how easy it looks, can be a challenge. It requires commitment and the support of certain attitudes or qualities of mind. It's like planting a tree: although your desire and motivation to make it grow might be there, without all the necessary factors present, the tree will not flourish.

In the same way, practicing mindfulness requires a strong foundation which is supported by the presence of seven attitudes. Work to cultivate these attitudes, so that you provide the right nourishment to your practice. You will discover that the attitudes are interdependent, so that when you deepen one, you strengthen them all.

Beginner's Mind. A beginner's mind helps you bring a fresh and curious attitude to each experience, no matter how familiar. This way of being is the essence of mindfulness. Be as a beginner in each situation, bringing curiosity and openness to the experience, as if experiencing it for the first time.

- *Patience.* Patience allows you to be immersed in each experience at your own pace, without rushing or forcing yourself to move faster. Just let the process unfold in its own time and be present in each moment.
- *Non-judging.* This attitide is central to mindfulness. Being nonjudgmental means calmly and objectively observing internal and external experience, and acknowledging it for what it is without labelling or judging it as right or wrong, good or bad, pleasant or unpleasant. It is what it is in any moment.
- *Non-striving.* With this attitude, you don't try to attain a goal, aim to feel a certain way, or achieve something special. You allow yourself to be in the present, with things as they are.
- *Trust.* When you trust yourself, you trust your own wisdom and innate goodness and you know to follow your own path, not anybody else's. After all, nobody knows you better than you know yourself.
- *Letting Go.* The attitude of letting go helps you relate to your experience with nonattachment. Our usual tendency is to want to hold onto experiences we like (grasping) or push away what we don't like (aversion). The practice of letting go helps release you from these tendencies so that you can be with things as they are, without getting caught.
- *Acceptance.* Finally, the attitude of acceptance of how things are is central to mindfulness. It doesn't mean being resigned; rather, it means accepting the situation for what it is, and seeing it clearly. This is often the first step toward change.

As you practice mindfulness, you cultivate and strengthen these seven attitudes. In turn, your mindfulness practice will flourish when these attitudes are present.

Don't do any task in order to get it over with. Resolve to do each job in a relaxed way, with all your attention. Enjoy and be one with your work.

—Thich Nhat Hanh

In her nursing blog post, *The Poetry of the IV*, Nurse Amanda Anderson's description of how she inserts an IV provides a good example of applying a mindful focus to what you might view as a mundane task. Approaching this task mindfully, in the way Anderson describes, can change the experience for both you *and* the patient. This is what she says:

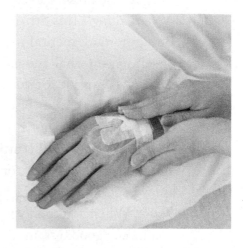

"I've been placing a lot of IVs lately…I've been working in the Cath Lab a lot, and we have a lot of elderly folks. Who don't have veins. And who hate needles… But even amidst the pressure, I've started taking a mental step back while I insert. I've started to crave a closer look at all of the various elements and sensations that come with starting an IV—the poetry of the process, if you will.

"The preparation is slightly ritualistic—just enough of the perfect collection of supplies (I no longer need a huge towel to catch blood—sometimes I don't spill a drop). The tourniquet, the way the patient's skin feels, the way their veins sometimes bulge and sometimes burrow—there is an order to the search. Success only comes with a certain quietness from within.

"Lately my favorite element has been the instant of insertion, the moment that I gently, slowly—no matter the din and chaos around me—communicate with the vein through the tip of my needle. It's like sewing a very delicate fabric; the slight upward motion of the needle going into the skin always surprises. What will the skin feel like against it? Will it be easy and smooth, or tough and resistant?

"Then, the tiniest of tiniest 'pops'—the needle entering the vein—how does one describe this? It is a feeling and an emotion—a letdown of relief and a moment of success and a confirmation of access all in one. There is no way to know it until you experience it...

"Now, IVs are a chance to chat—to talk with patients about where they live, what they do, how they feel. It's amazing how easy the moments become—even when I miss or blow a vein—if I focus on talking with people. I enjoy myself, the pressure lifts, and I assess them through our conversation. Patients bare deep wounds in these tiny moments.

"It is magical to provide access to a person's life force—their blood...There are days when I never miss a shot, others when I apologize more than gloat. But isn't this the process of nursing? One IV at a time."[12]

While Amanda inserts the IV, she is practicing "beginner's mind"—an attitude of openness and curiosity, a quality of awareness that relates to each experience as fresh and new. You can feel Amanda's sense of awe as she approaches the task of inserting the IV. Beginner's mind helps you disengage from your automatic way of doing things and approach each activity as though for the first time. Then, even the smallest and most ordinary moments shine.

Can you imagine approaching your life and work like that?

Journal Reflection:

Reflect for a moment on other attitudes that Amanda embodies as she inserts the IV. Which of these attitudes are present for you as you carry out your daily nursing tasks? Which attitude do you most need to cultivate? For the next eight weeks, practice a different attitude each week, and record your experience in your journal.

Let Go of Your Workday

Okay, you've made it through another shift, and you're on your way out the door. In no time, your mind races to the concerns waiting for you at home—*the future*—or to disturbing things that happened at work—*the past*. The result? You feel even more stressed, making it difficult to unwind once you get home. But now that mindfulness is your steady companion, you have the tools to turn this around. You can relax after a long day by entering the same state of *being* that you inhabited at the start of your shift.

Look out a window and find something to focus on, taking a moment to appreciate the experience of being part of the world around you. Sit still in the car or train and take a few breaths, feeling your abdomen expand and retract. Gently allow your attention to settle there, aware of the rhythm of the in-breath and out-breath. Leave work behind, letting go of all the responsibilities you had there. Your natural state is in the present moment.

Practice Plan:

This week, use mindful handwashing as your anchor activity, letting it be a time to de-stress and reconnect with yourself. As you go about your day, set the intention of cultivating beginner's mind while engaging with your colleagues and patients as well as your daily tasks.

For your formal practice, set aside fifteen minutes daily to practice mindfulness of breathing. Keep doing these practices until they become a natural part of your day. Record your experience in your journal.

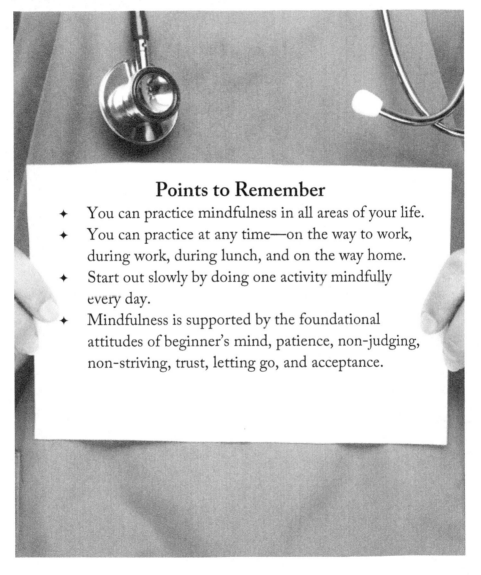

Points to Remember

+ You can practice mindfulness in all areas of your life.
+ You can practice at any time—on the way to work, during work, during lunch, and on the way home.
+ Start out slowly by doing one activity mindfully every day.
+ Mindfulness is supported by the foundational attitudes of beginner's mind, patience, non-judging, non-striving, trust, letting go, and acceptance.

CHAPTER FOUR

Reaping the Benefits of Mindfulness Practice

You have to actually practice mindfulness in order to reap its benefits and come to understand why it is so valuable.

—Jon Kabat-Zinn

Ultimately, mindfulness is a way of being that becomes more natural with practice. If you set aside time to practice it regularly, you do see the benefits—the more practice, the greater the effect.

Jean was a nurse practitioner in the emergency room. She had grown to hate her job and spent most of her work time wishing she were somewhere else. She felt stressed even at the *thought* of going to work. Mindfulness practice was a revelation for Jean and helped her see how much time she spent judging the moment she was in, and how unhappy that made her feel. She discovered that she could observe the judging mindfully and be curious about it, rather than getting lost in it. This allowed her to become increasingly aware of moments when she fought against how things were.

When she had to write orders for a new admit, she noticed that she braced herself against engaging with this tedious job. Her shoulders were tight, her jaw was clenched, and there was a knot in her stomach; she procrastinated as long as she could, which caused additional problems as the shift progressed. Once she became aware of these unpleasant sensations, she was able to breathe gently into them, and the sensations eventually subsided. Jean discovered that she could be present more often with her experience and accept rather than judge it or fight it. This helped her stop waiting until work was over to really live her life. As she began to live more in the here-and-now, she realized that her experience was actually okay. It was her resistance to it that was causing the problem!

> Submit to a daily practice.
> Your loyalty to that
> Is a ring at the door.
> Keep knocking, and the joy inside
> Will eventually open a window
> and look out to see who's there.
> —Rumi

Submit to a Daily Practice

Jean gave herself the gift of time and space every day to practice mindfulness, and she reaped the benefit of living a fuller life. Maybe you can you do the same by taking some time to step away from the hustle and bustle of everyday life just to *be*. In the same way you exercise to take care of your body, a daily mindfulness practice can help care for your mind.

Consider This:

Do you spend your waking hours obsessing about how you no longer enjoy your work? Do these thoughts keep you from focusing on your tasks? Do you get easily frustrated and edgy when your patient's needs change suddenly? Are you quick to judge yourself, others, or situations negatively, without taking the time to hear the whole story, or see the situation for what it really is?

Pick a timeslot that works for you, and bear in mind that, if you put it off until after a busy shift, it's likely you will nod off as soon as you close your eyes. The ideal time may be in the morning as soon as you wake up. Whatever time you choose, try to sit at that approximate time (e.g., morning or lunchtime) every day. That way, it will more easily become a habit.

Each day, take your seat for meditation, wherever is comfortable and reasonably quiet for you, and set your timer. Continue sitting until the timer goes off, no matter what comes up in your body or mind. More than likely, there will be an onslaught of thoughts about all the other things you should be doing. Just notice those thoughts and gently redirect your attention to your breath.

Once you've practiced for five minutes daily for a week or two, you can gradually stretch your practice to fifteen or twenty minutes. What is most important at the outset is that it becomes a habit.

When you are ready for a more serious commitment, you might pledge to work up to Kabat-Zinn's recommendation of forty-five minutes of meditation at least six days a week.

Benefits to Becoming More Mindful

Like Jean, you will experience many changes when you bring mindfulness into your everyday life. Perhaps you have already noticed some benefits. For example, have you noticed how doing everyday activities mindfully makes those activities more satisfying —how pleasant activities become even more pleasant when done mindfully, and unpleasant or stressful activities lose some unpleasantness when you approach them with openness and curiosity?

With continued practice, your physical and psychological well-being will improve. Equally important, you will be better able to respond to the stress in your life. Other benefits of mindfulness practice include:

🌿 *Improved Focus.* The practice of mindfulness sharpens your attention and focus. You become better equipped to cope with distractions and interruptions, which is no small feat in nursing!

🌿 *Positive Emotions.* Mindfulness practice boosts positive emotions while reducing stress and negative thoughts. In turn, this increases satisfaction with life both at home and at work.

🌿 *Decision-making.* Research suggests that even brief periods of mindfulness may improve decision-making skills.[13] As decision-making skills improve, patient safety and communication may also improve.

🌿 *Flexibility and Creativity.* Research has shown that observation skills and cognitive flexibility improve with mindfulness practice. As a result, you may notice solutions pop up where you never before thought to look for them and discover novel, creative ways around patient dilemmas.

🌿 *Emotion Regulation.* Regulating emotions becomes easier with mindfulness, helping you to respond rather than react, thereby improving communication and your relationships with others.

🌿 *Resilience.* Mindfulness builds resilience and facilitates the emotional stability required to be present for yourself and others.

🌿 *Compassion.* Research shows that kindness and compassion—for others and for oneself—are higher in people who practice mindfulness. Also, a positive side effect of kindness and compassion is an increase in happiness and well-being. We all learned as children that showing kindness and compassion is a good thing, but now we know that it's good for us, too!

Journal Reflection

From the practices you have tried so far, what benefits, if any, have you noticed in your own life? How much time and energy are you willing to commit to your daily practice?

Everybody Wins with Mindfulness

One very exciting finding has been that when you are mindful, your patients also benefit *directly*. How do we know this? In 2013, Dr. Mary Catherine Beach and her colleagues at Johns Hopkins University studied forty-five physicians, nurse practitioners, and physician assistants to see whether higher levels of mindfulness had an effect on patient/clinician encounters. Caregivers self-rated their levels of mindfulness using the Mindful Attention Awareness Scale (MAAS).

Interestingly, they discovered that even short encounters between mindful nurses and patients generated distinct positive effects. Those caregivers who reported higher levels of mindfulness typically enjoyed longer, more rewarding interaction with their patients and conveyed a more positive emotional tone.

The result? Patients forged emotional connections with these caregivers. They opened up about their difficulties and about what mattered to them. Just imagine how important, how pivotal, this could be for people from underserved or marginalized populations who might struggle to trust and feel respected by their healthcare providers. Think of how effective you could be in building such needed trust with these patients and the impact you could have on their well-being, not just now but going forward!

If you are worried that being mindful requires that you spend more time with each of your patients, don't be. Although the caregivers who reported high levels of mindfulness were admittedly more likely to spend more time with each patient, *that was not always the case*. Hence, increased patient satisfaction did not always require caregivers to spend more time with them.

This suggests that mindfulness alone—*regardless of the length of your patient interaction*—can noticeably enhance the quality of your encounter for both you and your patient. Even a short period of genuine and focused attention on your patient as a whole person can have positive effects.

Beach reported that such results might be due to how patients view both their condition and the level of quality in the care they receive, and that this perception affects the patients' healing process and overall sense of well-being.

In addition to bringing a more positive tone to patient encounters, mindful practitioners tended to *respond* rather than *react* to stressful situations. This increased their patients' confidence in them. It's a positive snowball effect.

Stressful Shifts

Every nurse has stressful shifts. And stress can push your buttons. Your emotions may be triggered by even simple challenges like patients refusing to take their prescribed medications, or refusing their ordered therapies.

Have you ever "lost it" during a stressful situation and then regretted it afterwards? Everyone reacts at times, but mindfulness helps you to notice reactivity as it builds. Then you can recognize and acknowledge feelings and thoughts—including anxious and fearful ones, as well as bodily tension—before they escalate, preventing yourself from reacting inappropriately.

You can then step back, unhook from the thinking that fuels the difficult emotions that threaten to spill over, and act from a wiser place. In a split second, a moment of mindfulness stops you from losing it and upsetting your patient.

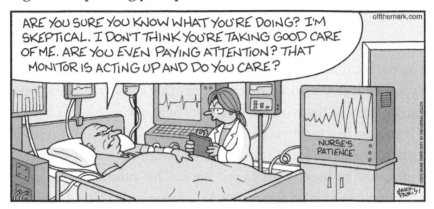

The more you learn to notice the accumulation of difficult thoughts, feelings, and bodily sensations, the better you can manage self-destructive urges and avoid acting on them.

Can you envision being unruffled by a sick patient's temper tantrum or calmly stepping up and doing what needs to be done in a code arrest when the people around you are panicked and confused? When you are calm and nonreactive, your patients, in turn, may find it easier to regulate their own difficult emotions. Sylvia Ford, an oncology nurse, finds that mindfulness helps her respond to the stresses she encounters every day at work, helping to set the emotional tone during a difficult situation and preventing it from escalating. "A few minutes of mindful breathing help calm my mind in the midst of a difficult situation. This helps me manage my stress levels and deal with challenging patients and coworkers as well as the hustle and bustle in my workplace," says Sylvia.

Cultivating Acceptance

Mindfulness doesn't change life. Life remains as fragile and unpredictable as ever. What changes is the heart's capacity to accept life as it is. It teaches the heart to be more accommodating, not by beating it into submission, but by making it clear that accommodation is a gratifying choice.

—Sylvia Boorstein

Think for a moment about your everyday experience. To what extent do you normally accept what is unfolding in the present moment? Are you like Jean whom we met earlier in this chapter, wishing your moments away so that you can be somewhere else?

If you are like most people, you spend a good portion of your day judging your experience in some way, wishing you were at the beach, a sports event, or home with a good book. This automatic tendency to judge propels us to push against, and to desire something other than, our current experience. If, on the other hand, our experience feels exactly like we want it to, we may cling to it and worry that it will change. These reactions are common to everyone.

Jean's habit of judging led to resistance—to the point where she found it challenging just to be at work. Fortunately, with practice, she was able to become aware of the judging and accept the moment as it was.

When you are mindful, you accept your experience for what it is rather than resisting it or clinging to it. As such, acceptance is an integral part of mindfulness. When you practice sitting meditation, you learn to be with and accept whatever arises in your awareness. This experience then carries into the rest of your day so you are more able to accept your inner experience as well as what happens in the course of your everyday life. Instead of dreading the next admission, the next code arrest, or thinking that the day will never end, take a few moments to appreciate where you are.

Acceptance doesn't mean you should become resigned to an unfair situation or that you shouldn't try to change things. Obviously, if you are uncomfortable and there is something you can do to improve the situation, by all means, do it. For example, if a visiting policy is unfair to families, it makes sense to think about how it can be changed and possibly proposing a trial to your manager. If you are unhappy in your job, there's no point putting up with unnecessary suffering. Make things better if you can, or leave if you need to. Nurses are usually out-of-the box thinkers, and that talent allows them to see what changes are required and what measures can be taken toward improvement.

It is often not possible, however, to change a situation you are in. For instance, you might find yourself in the midst of a very busy shift with a long list of things to do. You can't change that. In the end, you have two options: you can spend your time wishing it were different, or you can accept that this is how it is *right now*. Mindfulness helps you open up to things as they are and acknowledge your present-moment reality.

Does mindfulness mean you should put up with unfair working conditions? Absolutely not! Many healthcare organizations have started offering mindfulness to their staff, and this is a positive development. However, mindfulness should never be used as a band aid fix for unfair working conditions. As well as offering mindfulness, healthcare organizations must also make wider, systemic changes. Mindfulness may help empower you, as a nurse, to take mindful assertive action to address inequities in your workplace, rather than sit around waiting for change to happen. As you become mindful of what is going on within your healthcare organization, you may become more able to take wise action to address inequities and show compassionate concern.

Even when you're involved in a negative situation that you *can* change, a mindful attitude helps to ease the tension and move you through the challenge to a solution. It's stressful to make changes that other people may disapprove of, resist, or judge you for. A mindful attitude provides the stability you need to endure in peace until you've made things better.

The Three-Step Breathing Space

At times, work can feel overwhelming. When you need to recharge, practice pausing throughout your day. Try the following three-step breathing space practice the next time you have a break or get a few moments to duck away from the action.

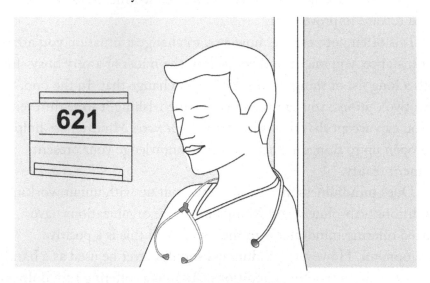

Try This:
The Three-Step Breathing Space

This practice involves three steps, each of which can take as little as a minute. If you don't have three minutes to devote to it, don't worry. Take whatever time you can. (You can access the guided audio recording of this practice by visiting www.nursingmindfully.com.)

Sit straight in a chair—not rigidly, but upright. If sitting is not an option, then stand. The idea is to tell your body that something is different, that you are setting the intention to be present.

Collect Your Awareness. Bring your awareness to your body. Do your feet hurt from standing all day? Does your back ache after lifting a patient? Perhaps you notice the feel of the coffee cup handle between your fingers or your body pressed against the chair.

Notice your thoughts and feelings. Are you feeling frustrated or angry? Relieved to be on break? Fidgeting because you are anxious to finish your list? Is your mind wandering to thoughts about a particular patient or coworker? Rather than judging what you are feeling or thinking, simply notice and allow it.

Gather Your Attention. Now that you are aware of what's happening in your experience, focus on the sensations in your abdomen as you breathe. If your mind wanders, gently bring it back.

Expand Your Awareness. Now, moving your attention outward from your abdomen to the rest of your body, notice your posture, adjusting it, if need be…becoming aware of your facial expression, allowing any tension there to fall away.

Notice the sensations of breathing throughout your body, feeling your whole body breathing, from your head down to your legs and feet, accepting any sensations as part of this complete, living, and breathing you.

Journal Reflection:

After you practice the breathing space, take a moment to reflect on what you noticed.

The breathing space is regarded as a formal rather than an informal practice, but because it takes so little time to do, you can practice it anytime once you've learned it. You don't have to sit in a special meditation spot. You can practice wherever and whenever you feel the need to pause and reconnect with the present moment. Think of all that time spent in the car, in the line at the grocery, waiting for a patient's treatment to finish…use those moments wisely!

If you find yourself saying, "I really need to meditate, but I just can't find the time," remember the three-step breathing space. It offers you a simple way to grow more comfortable with small moments of focused practice and makes it easier to progress to formal meditation practice.

Jacinta Clarke worked in the ICU step-down unit. She often reached the end of her workday with only a vague recollection of the day's events. It was as though she were on autopilot mode all the time, frantically racing from task to task. Sometimes she would think she still needed to administer patients their pain medicine, but when she looked at the computer, she'd realize she had already given it.

Things started to change for Jacinta shortly after she started the mindfulness course her facility hosted. For her, the three-step breathing space was the most useful practice she took away from the training. She was excited to discover that mindfulness didn't always take more time; it just required that she use her time a little differently.

Once Jacinta became familiar with the breathing space, she set the intention to practice it at regular intervals. The times she chose were before shift report, before patient rounds, and between routine tasks.

How did it change her day? "After doing the breathing space, I notice that I am not so stressed. It helps me let go of accumulated tension so I can move on to my next task in a way that is more relaxed, yet productive and clear-headed. I feel I can make a fresh start," Jacinta reports.

Every moment of your workday offers an opportunity to become present. If you make a generous commitment to daily formal practice, the benefits will seep into your nursing. You will be more grounded, focused, and tuned into what you're doing and what's going on around you. In the same way that you slot other appointments into your daily schedule, make room for mindfulness practice, too. Give it the same priority. Without doubt, you will reap the benefits from doing so.

Practice Plan:

Congratulations! You have reached the end of the first section of this book.

Take some time now to integrate the practices you have learned so far before you continue reading. Remember to bring the three-step breathing space into your daily routine and practice it at intervals throughout your day. Observe how these mindful pauses change your experience. Also continue to practice mindful breathing daily, supporting your practice with patience, acceptance, and the other foundational attitudes you have learned about.

What do you notice? In the course of your day, check in and observe how often you are preoccupied with liking or disliking your experience. Instead, set the intention to become aware of these judgments and of any changes in your experience as you do so. When you feel ready, pick up the book again and continue reading. Meanwhile, acknowledge yourself for the commitment you have made and the time you have invested in your mindfulness journey thus far!

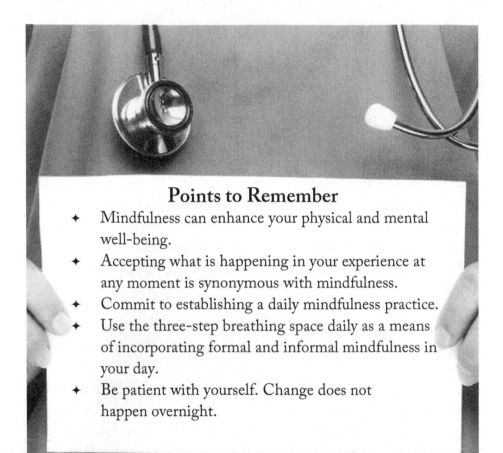

Points to Remember

+ Mindfulness can enhance your physical and mental well-being.
+ Accepting what is happening in your experience at any moment is synonymous with mindfulness.
+ Commit to establishing a daily mindfulness practice.
+ Use the three-step breathing space daily as a means of incorporating formal and informal mindfulness in your day.
+ Be patient with yourself. Change does not happen overnight.

PART II

MINDFULNESS AND THE BODY

Realize that this very body, with its aches and its pleasures…is exactly what we need to be fully human, fully awake, fully alive.

—Pema Chödrön

CHAPTER FIVE
Mindful Self-Care

Practicing within the epicenter of illness and loss, nurses must ensure
that their well-being is cultivated with the same rigor,
intensity, and expertise extended to those they nurse.

—*Self-Healing through Reflection,*
by Nancy Jo Bush and Deborah A. Boyle

The more you practice mindfulness and compassion, the more aware
you become of how you spend your time at work, at home, and
everywhere else. To begin the process of becoming self-aware, ask
yourself the following questions:

- *Am I taking average, good, or great care of myself in my everyday life?*
- *Am I treating myself with the same care and kindness I would show a good friend or a vulnerable patient?*
- *How often do I remember to take breaks, eat meals, use the bathroom, or drink enough water?*
- *How often do I slow down, pause, stretch, and take a deep breath?*

Rosaleen Fox was an operating room nurse. She worked
on telemetry for three years but was unhappy due to the short
staffing, management's failure to institute policies to help floor
nursing, and the entitlement many patients seemed to feel when
they came into the hospital. She was thrilled to be accepted for a
position in the operating room based on her former performance
on the telemetry unit.

The newness of her role made Rosaleen eager to go to work every day. She enjoyed taking care of her patients, assuring they came through surgery safely. Although her hours were still long, she looked forward to getting called in for a case. However, the longer she stayed with the unit, the more the old feelings of discontent resurfaced. She had to lift patients far more often than she did on the telemetry unit, and it took forever to get vital supplies and equipment to the room because it seemed there was never enough to go around.

Once again, over time, she grew to hate her job and to dread going to work. Even when she wasn't physically at work, her mind was still there. Often she would worry about dealing with a particular coworker or about not being able to find needed equipment. One day she had a meltdown in the lunchroom and was mortified that her manager witnessed it.

The manager suggested Rosaleen see a therapist through the facility's employee assistance program. Although Rosaleen wasn't convinced a therapist would help, she went anyway. To her surprise, she gained a tremendous amount of insight into her problem through therapy.

Rosaleen learned quickly that the unit she was on was not the problem. Rather, her pattern of ignoring her own needs was making her hate her job, and her attitude toward the job, as well as her lack of self-care, led to feelings of anger, depression, and apathy.

Consider This:

Do you skip meals at work, or rush through them, without properly chewing? Do you end up with stomach upsets after your meals? Do you finish your shift with a full bladder? Is your mind still at work when you are at home, and on days off?

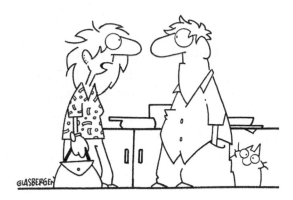

"I was so tired at work, the other nurses had to revive
me with C.P.R. — Coffee, Pepsi, and Redbull!"

Just as you offer advice on self-care to your patients, you can—
and should—offer that same kindness to yourself. In fact, you need
to learn how to care for yourself before you can properly care for your
patients. Otherwise, you may well end up depleted, like Rosaleen.

By examining the wisdom of the body, you can see a profound
model of self-care in the way the heart first perfuses itself, before
pumping blood to vital organs like the brain, the lungs and the rest
of the circulatory system. If the heart didn't perfuse itself first, we
wouldn't survive the daily stressors of life.

Mindfulness helps you develop self-awareness and find balance.
When you are mindful, you quickly become alert to those minutes,
hours, and days when you're not taking great care of yourself. Regular
practice helps you listen to your body, and in time you learn to
improve the relationship you have with yourself, which is central to
self-care.

Mindfulness of Daily Activities

As you practice mindfulness daily, the *quality* of your days may
change. You will find more harmony and ease, coupled with less
stress and distraction.

Try This:
Mindful Daily Activities

The following simple exercise comes from the Mindfulness-Based Cognitive Therapy (MBCT) curriculum.[14] MBCT is quite similar to MBSR, and this exercise is designed to help you become more aware of how you spend your time.

Close your eyes and imagine a typical day. See yourself moving through the hours and minutes from the moment you wake up. What are the kinds of things you typically do? Take your time when reflecting on this, and when you're ready, open your eyes.

Make a list of all the activities that came to mind. The following might appear on your list: taking a shower, getting dressed, having breakfast, going for a run, driving to work, assessing patients, looking over doctors' orders, gathering supplies, going to lunch, meeting a friend, checking Facebook, going to the grocery store, reading a book or magazine. Circle the top twelve activities you engage in most regularly.

Next to each activity, write either an "N" or a "D." Mark "N" for activities you find nourishing and "D" for activities you find draining. Nourishing activities energize and uplift you, while draining activities deplete your energy. If an activity on your list is neither, then record it as neutral (0). Some activities on your list may be both nourishing *and* draining. If that's the case, then record both N and D next to the activity. If you're unsure, take the time to notice what sensations and emotions are present the next time you do that activity.

Now look at your list. What do you notice? How even is the balance between nourishing and depleting activities? Do you sometimes resist doing the very things, such as eating breakfast or taking time to exercise, that nourish you and give you energy?

Journal Reflection:

Take a moment to reflect on what you have learned from the previous exercise. Is there anything in your routine that you would like to change? Perhaps you could find more time to do nourishing things or become more aware of them. For instance, can you allot fifteen minutes a day to meditate, making it part of your nourishing routine? Can you reduce the number of draining activities? Even if you can't reduce the number or frequency of depleting activities, could you bring a different attitude to these activities or make an adjustment of some kind? For instance, perhaps you could leave for work each day a little earlier, opening up space to enjoy a stress-free drive.

Nurse Sandra Jones learned how small adjustments in her daily routine can lessen stress. Sandra worked as a flight nurse for the local medical transport company. Although she enjoyed her work, the sight of so many victims of motor vehicle crashes and crime made her feel sad for all the suffering in the world. To find something outside of work that could distract her from the overwhelming parts of her job, Sandra decided to take a class at her local college. She couldn't find anything of interest, so she took a mindfulness class, even though she really had no idea what it was about.

As Sandra progressed through the course, she began to notice the unnecessary strain she caused herself by populating her day with depleting activities. She realized that, while she was always on the go, she didn't really enjoy anything as she rushed from task to task. Although Sandra knew she couldn't drop any activities on her list, she realized she could make some small but significant changes. For example, instead of pacing in the call room or mindlessly reading an entertainment magazine while she waited for the next transport request, she took the time for a mindful pause. Those few moments of mindful breathing nourished her, and she was able to be fully present when she responded to the next emergency. During a flight, when her patient's condition had stabilized, she practiced loving-kindness meditation, wishing for the person's good health and recovery. Afterwards, instead of mindlessly performing the downtime task of restocking the helicopter, she challenged herself to pay close attention to the labels, expiration dates, and correct par levels before moving on. Then, at the base, she took time to eat lunch at her leisure, appreciating the food and enjoying a break from the busyness of her day. Sandra began to use these little moments as opportunities to come off autopilot mode and reconnect with herself. As she continued to make small changes in the way she approached her daily tasks, she felt less hurried and gained more appreciation for her job and the difference she could make in the life of her patients. Her feeling of accomplishment in a job well done, combined with the knowledge that her patients benefitted from her mindful focus, renewed her energy and focus.

The Need for Peace and Quiet

Even if your unit does not see trauma victims like Sandra's medical evacuation company, every hospital has its share of chaos. Let's face it: hospitals are not peaceful places to work. Between the demands of patients in need, the questions of colleagues, and the constant buzzing and beeping of technology—including your own cell phone—your days are probably filled with noise and activity.

How can you find peace and quiet in the midst of chaos?

Try This:
Mindful Steps
Count your steps as you walk down the hall. Pay attention to your breath and your footsteps, and let the rest go. You'll be surprised at how such a simple thirty-second exercise can help.

Everyone needs quiet time, and you are no exception. If you leave work feeling ragged and exhausted, the solution is to search for small moments of peace and quiet during your day. Take every opportunity to drop out of *doing* and slip into *being* mode. This can change the shape of your interactions with patients, families, colleagues, and with yourself. Although it sometimes takes a while to break old habits, it will be well worth the time you invest.

Journal Reflection:

Ask yourself these critical questions:

How do you know when you need a break from the hustle and bustle?

Can you make small (or big) changes to avoid overstimulation?

What would help you to do this?

The Need for Balance

We all know what it feels like to be out of balance. Whether it's physical, mental, or emotional imbalance, the symptoms typically include irritability, achiness, exhaustion, and frustration. The more mindful you become, the more you will notice your mind and body rebalancing.

To experiment with finding your balance, try the following practice that has roots in yoga and tai chi.

Try This:
Mindful Balance

Stand with your feet apart, each foot directly beneath the corresponding hip. Slowly rock back and forth, from right to left, foot to foot, until the rocking becomes almost imperceptible as you find your balance.

How long did it take to find your balance? How does balance in your physical body translate into balance in your work life and personal life? In your thoughts and feelings?

Self-care is never a selfish act. It is simply good stewardship of the only gift I have, the gift I was put on earth to offer to others.

—Parker Palmer

Restorative Pauses

In the same way you manage your time or your finances, it is important to manage your energy. Fortunately, this doesn't have to involve a lot of time or money. Instead, it's all about the little things.

What little things can you do to restore your energy? You might choose to walk slowly and mindfully down the corridor rather than racing. Maybe you can take a moment to look at a picture of loved ones, or look out the window and appreciate the view. You can joke around with a coworker, read a quote that inspires you, or ask a patient about family or hobbies. Simple things go a long way toward making your work and personal life more mindful and enjoyable.

While long pauses, like a weeklong tropical vacation, can certainly be blissful and restorative, sometimes the little breaks mean the most. How often do you simply rest—not sleep, but pause to rest? Even though a restful pause can change the shape of your day and

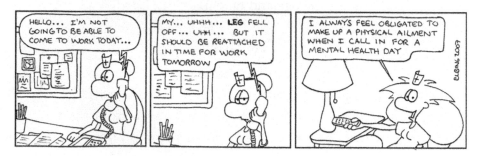

make work and energy flow more freely, like most people, you may find it difficult to do nothing, even for a few minutes.

Can you build restorative pauses into your day? Try getting into the habit of pausing for a few seconds every time you complete a task, before you move on to the next activity.

Ursula Walsh, a nurse who works nights in the telemetry unit at her local hospital, describes mindfulness as an essential part of her self-care plan: "It gives me space and time for a daily pause where I can check in with myself. Before, my body was in one place while my mind was scurrying off somewhere else. Now I feel more at home in myself. Even in the midst of a hectic shift, I know I can always pause and connect with the calm, balanced part of me that is always here, no matter how noisy, busy, or pressured things are on the outside."

Caring for Your Feet

Your feet are complex body parts that serve you well. Each foot has twenty-eight muscles and a miraculous lattice of tendons that work in harmony to bring about the engineering feat called walking. The process is so sophisticated that it takes years to develop the skills needed to stand, balance, initiate and stop movement, jump, and run.

Unfortunately, your job can make it easy to abuse and neglect your feet until they throb and ache. Standing for hours on hard surfaces can be painful, and feet that aren't regularly cared for will start to degrade. Further, neglecting to care for your feet can set up a domino effect of imbalance in your body. Sore feet will send ripples of pain up your spine, and you may end up slouching, balancing your weight unevenly, or developing blisters.

Try This:
Mindful Foot Care

Take time to rest your feet throughout the day. Stretch them regularly to release built-up tension. Wiggle your toes to boost blood flow, then shake your feet and rotate your ankles. Take a moment to stand up straight, feet planted, with your weight evenly distributed.

At the end of the day, as part of your de-stress ritual, soak your feet in hot water and try rubbing them down. Why not invest in an aromatherapy foot scrub and lotion?

Even better, treat yourself to a professional foot massage every now and then.

Most important of all, be sure to invest in proper, supportive footwear, and replace worn shoes.

When you practice mindful self-care, you feel more comfortable on your feet. Your patients benefit, too, since they receive better care when you can move about more comfortably, free from being distracted by lower-back pain or blisters.

Hydration, Urination, and the UTI

Most nurses joke about it, but urinary tract infections are no laughing matter. If you go through your entire shift without taking in a drop of liquid or, more importantly, emptying your bladder, you risk a urinary tract infection.

When you don't drink enough water, you inevitably become dehydrated, and your thinking may be affected. Then you are also more likely to feel tired and less able to concentrate. One way to prevent this is to keep a water bottle on your desk and drink regularly during the day.

During a busy shift, you might ignore or not even notice that your bladder is full. You've been too busy reacting to one situation after another to pay attention. If you take a moment to stop and tune in to your body, you might discover that you need to use the bathroom.

Some nurses convince themselves that they don't have time to think of themselves during busy shifts. This is understandable, but it isn't always true. You may be able to pass off your patients to a coworker for the five minutes it will take to get a drink of water or empty your bladder. When you return, you could offer to do the same for your coworker. Just like you, your coworkers may not have given any thought to their need to take a break, so by offering, you can help them to become more aware of their needs.

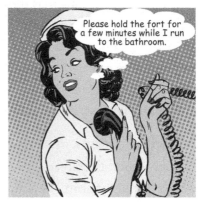

As a nurse, you know that research shows that ignoring your hydration and bodily functions often leads to chronic infections, incontinence, prostrate inflammation, and even kidney damage. So why put yourself at risk when some simple lifestyle changes can help you avoid all of that?

Graham Newell, a retired nurse, put it this way: "It is imperative that nurses take breaks, without question. Many harried nurses insist they don't have time to do so, but the more savvy and experienced nurses don't work without them. Nurses can't take care of others unless they take care of their own needs. It wasn't until I began to suffer with serious health issues related to poor eating habits that I realized how detrimental it was to neglect my own needs to eat and use the bathroom regularly. I would be healthier today if I had taken the time to be mindful of my own needs."

When you feel you have no time, take a deep breath. Remember that you can't care for anyone else until you care for yourself.

Journal Reflection:

How mindful are you of your body's needs during your shift? Do you stay hydrated and use the bathroom when you need to?

Grace Williams, a nurse practitioner assigned to the cardiothoracic surgery specialty, finds that the biggest change for her since she started practicing mindfulness is that she now takes her breaks. "Even when I'm really busy, I notice when I'm hungry or I need to use the bathroom. I no longer ignore my own needs. I'm more assertive, able to set limits, and say *no* when I need to, and my colleagues respect me for it. When I mind myself and take my breaks, my work actually improves."

Mindful Sleep

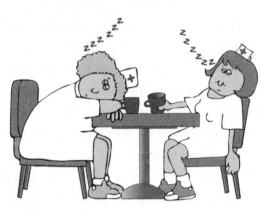

Nurses, especially those who work night shifts or staggered schedules, often struggle with sleep issues. Sooner or later, lack of sleep can lead to frustration and illness, and poor sleep can cause a wide range of mental and physical health issues.

People who practice mindfulness find that their sleep quality tends to improve. To make your bedtime routine more mindful, try to go to bed around the same time every night. In general, follow the same ritual before going to sleep (such as washing your face, brushing your teeth, stretching, reading, and relaxing in bed). Avoid the TV, computer/tablet, or other stimulating media close to your bedtime since these activities can interfere with relaxation, even those seemingly harmless and mindless game apps like solitaire! Research has shown that when you read on a tablet or smart phone for a couple of hours before bedtime, your sleep may be delayed by about an hour.[15]

Once you have pulled up the covers, try to let go of any tension that has built up during the day. If you've had a few sleepless nights, do your best to let that go as well. Focusing on the fear that you will be unable to sleep only makes it harder to relax and rest. Instead, focus on your breathing. Be still and breathe in and out until you drift away. Much like counting sheep, this keeps your mind in the present.

The next morning you will be well-rested and have more energy for work—and the other aspects of your day.

Nourish Yourself

You spend your days taking care of others; you need to nourish yourself, too, and with whatever nurtures you best.

Nourishment comes in many forms. Nourishment can mean your mom's homemade soda bread, a walk with your best friend, or a snuggle with your dog.

Developing positive self-care is important, especially if you have been focusing too much on others or suffer from compassion fatigue. Whatever it is that you enjoy, that makes you feel nourished, start making time for it today!

Practice Plan:

Continue to practice sitting meditation for at least fifteen minutes daily and to use the breathing space at intervals during your day. Whenever you can, take a moment to clear your schedule of the things that make you feel tense or tired. Watch less television. Learn to say no to the people and things that bring you down. Instead, take that class you've been hoping to attend, or read the book that's been sitting on your nightstand for the past two years. Soak up some sunshine or get together with your fellow nurses after your shift. Your time is precious, so it makes sense to use it wisely.

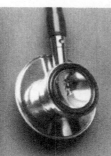
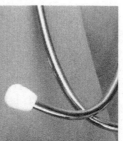

Points to Remember

✦ You need to learn how to care for yourself before you can care for your patients.

✦ Take small mindful breaks throughout your day to help focus on balance and self-care.

✦ Tune in to your body's needs. Stay hydrated and use the bathroom when you need to.

✦ To ensure you get a good night's sleep, make your bedtime routine more mindful, and follow that ritual each night.

CHAPTER SIX

Inhabiting Your Body

Many of us have not had enough practice in listening to our bodies.
The body is our first home. We can't feel at home in the outside world
if we're not at home in our own bodies.

—Thich Nhat Hanh

When you trained to become a nurse, you learned to understand and interact with other people's bodies. You learned to look at physical signs and symptoms, and to translate them into medical terms. In the same way, you recognized how distress and illness take shape in the body.

But how aware are you of your own body? In order to feel at home in the outside world and be present in the moment, you must first feel at home in your own flesh.

This was the experience of Rose, a former mindfulness student of mine. Rose had recently earned her RN license, having worked as an LPN for a long time. She decided to apply for a job in the heart cath lab. She knew what the job required when she started—she would be on her feet for twelve-hour shifts and would have to be prepared to attend to patients' needs before, during, and after the cath procedures. Sometimes she could barely breathe, keeping up with the volume of patients that came through the lab and the high-pressure stakes of possibly losing a patient. Those with multiple blockages required long procedures and were at a higher risk for complications or even death.

By the end of a shift, Rose would have to urinate so badly her bladder ached. After taking care of that emergency, the hunger she had been suppressing throughout her shift made its case for her attention. She would be so busy during her shifts that she seldom thought of her body's needs, or she ignored them so she could keep up with the pace in the lab. In any event, she would not let her body's needs get in the way of her work. It was almost as though Rose didn't have a body.

Consider This:

How often have you finished a shift feeling lightheaded and realized it was because you had forgotten to eat? Is your bladder so full at the end of a shift that it actually hurts to pee? Do you cringe in pain when you wash your hands because the skin is dry and cracked, even bleeding? Are you constantly breaking nails during care tasks?

Do you tune out your body's needs during your shifts, as Rose did? If you tune *in* to your body, you will become more aware of its needs and feel more focused. In turn, you will have better resources to help

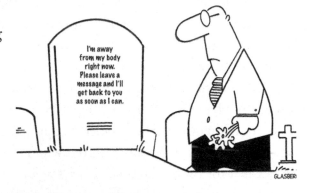

you survive the daily whirlwind of your work life—and become more available to your patients. This chapter will help you become mindful of your body and its needs, whatever they are and whenever they occur.

Get in Touch with Your Body

The Irish poet John O'Donohue remarked on how amazing it is that so many people are walking around in bodies, but without experiencing themselves bodily.[16] Your body is a living, breathing organism constantly responding to its environment. If your shift is particularly busy, you may forget all about your body and become disconnected from your immediate physical experience. The busier you are, the harder it is to stay in touch with your body and how it feels.

Like your mind, your body is not static. Although you may not notice it, your body's physical sensations shift constantly. Tuning in to your physical sensations grounds you in your body and anchors you in the moment. Take a few moments to notice what is happening in your body right now.

Try This:
Mindful Check-in

Can you sense how tense or relaxed your body feels?

How fast or slow is your breathing?

Do you feel hungry or satisfied? Alert or sleepy? Hot or cold?

Are your hands clenched shut or open and relaxed?

Do your shoulders feel tight or are they loose?

Is your body warm or cool? Is your skin prickling or relaxed?

Are you sitting still or shifting in your seat?

Tune in to any other sensations in your body. Do you feel pressure, hardness, softness, vibration, itching, tingling, pulsation, numbness?

Feel how the edges of your body define you. Notice whether you feel grounded or out of touch with the edges of your body.

Tune in to any odors or tastes you are experiencing as well as the sights and sounds around you. Be aware of what you are touching and of what touches your skin.

How was it to pause and notice how your body feels?

The body is the gateway to the present. When you check in to your body's sensations in this way, you come back to the present moment.

This kind of attention helps the body relax, and protects you from getting caught up in over-thinking. Set the intention to pause for a few seconds, at intervals throughout the day, and tune in to your body. Let's look at practices that will help you to do just that, so you can re-inhabit your body and anchor yourself in its stability.

Mindful Hands

When you practice nursing, you lend your hands to those in need. Think about it. Could you practice the art of nursing without the ability to gently feel for veins, lift patients from their beds, or hold another person's hand? In other words, could you nurse without your sense of touch?

Your hands translate your thoughts into action and communicate your intentions. For example, anger—even when you try to conceal it—can show itself in how tightly you clench your hands and your body. You might hurt patients by rushing through a procedure or handling them a little impatiently.

Hesitancy, on the other hand, manifests in a shaky, unsure touch, while distraction appears in hands that touch without really touching. Although your interaction may be wordless, a patient can feel your intention through your touch alone.

Do you use your hands as instruments of care and tenderness? Are you deliberate in your actions, careful and diligent, respecting the body you are touching? In the end, are you hurried and inattentive, or do your hands communicate warmth and compassion? This practice will help you to reconnect to your hands.

Try This:
Mindful Hands

Take a quiet moment to turn your attention to your hands...resting them in your lap, turning them slowly to see all dimensions and angles...noticing the weight of your hands and the creases and folds in the skin...noticing each of your fingers: the shape, color, and texture of your skin.

Open and close your palms slowly, noticing how your hands feel as they move...becoming aware of the exquisitely tiny and precise movements your hands can make...becoming aware of the temperature of your hands. Is your skin dry? Soft? Warm? Damp? Cool?

Reflect for a moment on the power you have in your hands. They are an expression of your care, the point at which your body reaches out and conveys compassion for others.

What's easy about this practice is that you can do it at any time during the day—when using public transportation, waiting for someone, or whenever ten minutes of time opens up in your schedule.

Journal Reflection:

How was this practice for you?

What did you notice?

How aware are you of your hands as you do your daily tasks?

Take some time to appreciate your hands, giving gratitude for all the work that they do. Enjoy this beautiful blessing of the hands from In Praise of Hands, by Diann Neu:[17]

> *Blessed be these hands that have touched life.*
> *Blessed be these hands that have felt pain.*
> *Blessed be these hands that have embraced with compassion.*
> *Blessed be these hands that have clenched with anger or*
>   *withdrawn in fear.*
> *Blessed be these hands that have drawn blood and*
>   *administered medicine.*
> *Blessed be these hands that have cleaned beds and disposed*
>   *of wastes.*
> *Blessed be these hands that have anointed the sick and*
>   *offered blessings.*
> *Blessed be these hands that grow stiff with age.*
> *Blessed be these hands that have comforted the dying and held*
>   *the dead.*
> *Blessed be these hands that hold the promise of the future.*

The Body Scan

Here is another practice that helps to ground your attention in the present by bringing your awareness to the body. But in this practice, rather than focusing on a single aspect of your physicality (such as the hands), you extend attention to the entire body and become aware of any sensations throughout. Although you may find yourself relaxing during the body scan, this is not the goal. Much time in the course of your everyday life may be lost in worrying, judging, and planning. The body scan helps quiet this running monologue of mental preoccupations, enabling you to shift into *being* mode and to notice sensations, including any points of stress or discomfort. Your usual response to bodily discomfort may be to numb it or to distract attention from it. By practicing the body scan, you learn instead to be present with these uncomfortable sensations, and bring a friendly awareness, acceptance, and curiosity to whatever is present, even when it is difficult or painful.

Try This:
Body Scan

Allow at least thirty minutes for the body scan. (To access a guided audio recording of this practice, visit www.nursingmindfully.com.)

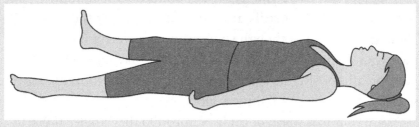

Turn off your phone and try to eliminate other potential distractions. Wear comfortable, loose-fitting clothes. The most comfortable position is to lie flat on your back, arms by your sides, palms facing up, and legs resting slightly apart. If necessary, support your neck or lumbar area with a pillow or folded towel. If lying down feels too uncomfortable, sit in a chair instead.

Give yourself permission to devote this time fully to you—to nourish yourself and receive whatever restoration the practice offers you. This time is not about changing things for the better or lamenting about what has slipped away. Accept relaxation if it happens without striving for it, because striving to relax may simply create more tension.

Let these steps guide you through the body scan.

(cont'd)

To begin, feel your body's weight, noticing the contact your body makes with the surface on which you are resting… noticing physical sensations in each body part: tingles, warmth, or tightness in any of your limbs… setting the intention to welcome whatever you encounter, whether it's emotional or physical.

When you become aware of intense sensations or tension anywhere in the body, use the in-breath to gently bring awareness into the sensations, and, on the out-breath, have a sense of the sensations releasing. This is called "breathing into" the sensation or body part.

Center on where you feel your breath the most, in the abdomen, chest or nostrils, resting your awareness there for some time…then, as though your awareness were a warm laser, pass your attention over your entire body…having a sense of your breath moving down to the toes of your left foot, taking with it any strain and tightness along the way.

Are your toes warm or cold? Numb? Do they tingle? If you're not noticing any sensation, be aware of the absence of feeling.

Move from the toes, to the ball, sole, and the heel of your foot…moving up around the sides, noticing any physical sensations, onto the top of the foot and up to the ankle…letting your foot slip from your awareness, moving your attention up into your left leg, noticing any heaviness, weight, or movement.

Now, releasing your left leg from your awareness, and roll your attention over and all the way down your right leg, ending at the toes…repeating the same process as before, coming up your right leg…, moving on from the leg to your pelvis, noting whether the sensations are pleasant or unpleasant as well as your reactions to them…as you leave each major area, breathing into it on the in-breath, then releasing that body part when you exhale.

(cont'd)

Bring your attention to your lower abdomen, observing how it rises and falls with each breath. Remain centered here for a moment, acknowledging any feelings and thoughts, noticing what is pleasant, unpleasant, or neutral in your experience...moving beyond the abdomen to your chest, noticing your rib cage as it moves with your breath...being aware of your heartbeat and how it works with the rest of your body to sustain life...shifting your awareness to your arms, noticing your wrists, forearms, elbows, and shoulders, and gradually feeling your breath flow into your hands...noticing the place where your spine meets your neck...moving your focus around to your face, observing each part of your mouth: the lips and tongue, all around the inside of the mouth...moving across the rest of your face...expanding awareness to your entire body, feeling your breath renew every muscle, bone, organ, and cell.

Lie still, breathing naturally, taking your time to linger here, feeling complete. As you end this practice, set the intention to bring any benefits with you as you move into the rest of your day.

Journal Reflection:

Take a little time now to reflect on your experience.

What did you notice during the body scan?

Were you aware of any pleasant or unpleasant sensations?

Did you notice your attention wandering?

How did you feel after doing the body scan?

Angela's Experience: Within minutes of lying down on her yoga mat for the body scan, Angela, a nurse in the mental health unit, was fast asleep. Working twelve-hour shifts three days a week was taxing.

Many patients on her unit would act out, and Angela felt as though she were trying to solve thirty problems at once. During the body scan, she decided to be kind to herself and simply enjoy the rest it offered. Clearly, she was exhausted. Angela knew the purpose of the body scan wasn't to fall asleep but to tune into the body's sensations. After a week of the practice, she decided to sit upright in a chair to help her stay awake and get the full benefit. Then she no longer nodded off, but her mind hopped from thought to thought. Should she tell her manager that the short staffing was stressing her out? Should she move to a floor that wasn't so emotionally taxing? Should she get a new car or try to keep the old one running? Angela felt frustrated. She had hoped the body scan would help clear her mind, but it felt like her mind was now busier than ever. Not only that, but she also became aware of aches and pains she had never noticed before.

Angela's experience is not unusual. In everyday life, your attention can easily be swept away in the stream of thoughts. During the body scan, you gently bring your attention back, no matter how often it wanders. Over time, regular practice helped Angela recognize areas of her body where she held tension. Her mind continued to wander, but less so, as she tuned into parts of her body under constant physical strain. Learning to breathe into these areas of discomfort reduced the negative effects of stress and helped her feel more at home in her body.

Ideally the body scan should be practiced every day over a period of weeks to sharpen your ability to pay attention. The full practice may take anywhere from twenty-five to forty-five minutes, although it's also possible to do it in less time, depending on your mood and schedule.

You can do a short body scan in as little as four minutes, anywhere and anytime, but it is particularly useful when you're feeling anxious or stressed. In no time at all, you will notice the rebalancing effects of this short practice. The process for the short body scan is the same as for the longer practice and can be done sitting, standing, or lying down.

Try This:
Short Body Scan

Bring your attention to the breath moving in your body.

Beginning with your feet, gradually move your attention up through your body, noticing sensations along the way…paying particular attention to areas where you tend to hold tension—perhaps your jaw, lower back, and shoulders…breathing into each area as you scan it, releasing any tension on the out-breath…gradually, expanding your awareness to the whole body, spending a few moments being aware of it, and of the breath flowing freely through it.

When to Do the Short Body Scan

You can get into the habit of doing short body scans in the midst of your regular activities. Here are some points in your day that may be especially conducive to the practice:

- when you end one activity and before you start another
- while sitting at the nurse's station
- while waiting on hold on the phone
- during lunch breaks
- before logging into the computer
- when you step onto your unit
- after receiving report
- before a procedure, such as an IV start
- after leaving a patient's room
- in your car after your shift

Mindfulness of Sounds

Stop reading for a moment, and listen to the sounds around you. What did you hear? Too often in life, we become lost in thought and unaware of what is going on inside and around us. Listening to sounds can help direct attention away from thoughts and back to what is happening here and now. Mindful listening brings you back to the present. If you work in a busy, noisy healthcare facility, there is likely to be a multitude of sounds, including beeps, alarms, and ringing phones to name but a few. Since many of these sounds possibly stress and irritate you, you might cope by tuning them out. However, paying attention to them instead can reduce the irritation. Notice how your body and mind react to a particular sound such as an alarm going off. There might be clenching in your stomach and shoulders, as well as thoughts such as "I don't like this." Once you become aware of these reactions, and take a moment to breathe with them, the tension softens. You will then be able to hear sounds without getting caught up in liking or disliking them. (To access a guided audio recording of mindfulness of sounds, visit www.nursingmindfully.com.)

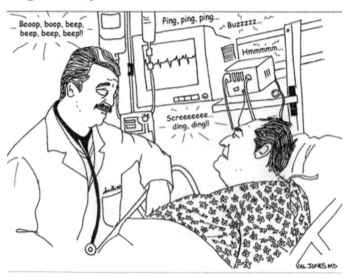

"These machines sure are life-savers, doc.
The noise annoyed me right out of my coma."

Try This:
Mindfulness of Sounds

Sitting up straight, allowing your body to be relaxed yet alert.

Focus on your breathing, and when you feel ready, bring your attention to hearing sounds.

Have a sense of your ears as satellites picking up sounds around you, noticing sounds in the far distance, such as traffic or airplanes, as well as more immediate sounds, outside or inside the room. Are there quiet humming sounds that you hadn't noticed? Is the wind blowing? Is it raining?

Be aware of sounds as sound waves that your body is receiving, noticing any stories, labels, or images that arise and letting them go…noticing where your attention is right now. If it's wandered away from sounds into thoughts about the past or future, gently bring it back to the soundscape around you.

Notice now if there's a sense of liking or disliking certain sounds…being aware of how the sound comes first, followed by liking or disliking. Just notice this, the interpretation or judgment that is added, and allowing it to be as it is.

If you become continuously distracted by a thought, an emotion, or body sensation, try labeling it. For example, "cramping…cramping." Or "worrying… worrying." Simply label and then gently return your attention to sounds, becoming aware of your emotional response to particular sounds. If there is tension or irritation, gently breathing with it...noticing how sounds appear and disappear…gradually bringing your attention back to the breath, focusing here for a few breaths… allowing your eyes to open gently, slowly bringing your attention into the room.

Journal Reflection:

How was your experience?

What sounds did you hear?

What reactions did you notice in your body and mind as you focused on sounds?

Bring this practice into your workday and tune in to the soundscapes that surround you. Listen to sounds as they come in and out of your awareness: the regular, mechanical puffs of a ventilator; the clock ticking; the shift change bustle at the nurses' station; and the squeak of wheels as a gurney goes down the hall. Be aware that the mind tends to create images, associations, and stories about the sounds we hear. Notice when this happens, and gently let these stories go, bringing your attention back to noticing sounds.

In the course of your workday, pay attention to how you register certain sounds as pleasant, unpleasant, or neutral. Notice how you react to each sound, feeling the sensations in your body. Do certain sounds, such as the beeping of the IV pump or the blare of a fall alarm induce frustration, tension, or anxiety? Can you let the reactivity fall away and just hear sounds as sounds?

Notice how you register the sounds that follow and how you react to them. Mark them with "P" for pleasant, "U" for unpleasant, and "N" for neutral:

- ☐ *Call bell ringing*
- ☐ *Blare of the fall alarm*
- ☐ *Telephone ringing*
- ☐ *Patient's call for help*
- ☐ *Blare of the television*
- ☐ *Beeping of high-tech machines*
- ☐ *Hum of the ventilator*

- ☐ *Wheezing breath sounds*
- ☐ *Crash cart rumbling down the hall*
- ☐ *Squeak of new shoes on linoleum*
- ☐ *Code blue claxon on the overhead speaker*
- ☐ *Patient crying*
- ☐ *Chatter of the next shift as they come down the hall*
- ☐ *Steady rhythm of an apical heart rate*
- ☐ *Patient saying "thank you"*
- ☐ *Clack of the keys on a keyboard*
- ☐ *Medications arriving via pneumatic tube*
- ☐ *Intercom announcements*

Walking Meditation

At work, not only are you surrounded by lively and noisy soundscapes, you are most likely on your feet and moving constantly. You walk up and down corridors, head to other departments from the nurses' station, pick up supplies, and make your rounds. Research has shown that the average nurse walks at least three miles during a regular shift, often up to five miles on a day shift.[18] Obviously, the size of your nursing unit and the nurse-to-patient ratio influence the distance you walk.

How much do you walk during an average shift? Do you spend this time on autopilot? If so, there is a way to turn this around. Think of walking not as an exercise in drudgery or a means to an end but as an opportunity to be mindful.

Instead of feeling your body as dead space, zoom in on what is happening minute by minute. Focus, in turn, on the powerful muscles in your legs that enable you to walk. So many tiny miracles of bioengineering unfold inside us at each given moment. Take every opportunity to notice what's going on in your body as you ambulate.

Try This:
Informal Walking Meditation

Focus, one at a time, on how your feet, legs, and spine feel, leaning into the sensation of weight and balance, noticing the rhythm of your body's movement, how your weight shifts, how your center of gravity swings with each new step and resettles across the surface of your feet...noticing the feeling of your feet on the floor, the sound of your shoes making contact with the floor... being aware of areas of tension or relaxation in your body as you walk.

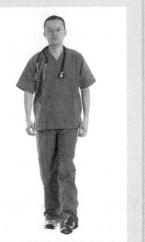

Build walking meditation into your day, when making rounds or moving from one room to another. When you go up and down stairs, use that time to practice. Even in the noisiest environment, you can still practice mindful walking.

Connor Allen, a nurse on a medical-psych unit, describes his experience of mindful walking: "Just ten minutes of walking meditation restores me. When the ward is quiet, I take the opportunity to practice a simple walking meditation. I concentrate on feeling my feet touching the floor as I walk the corridor, going from room to room. These short breaks help clear my mind. I do longer walking meditations on my days off work. My favorite is when I take an early morning walk along the road that runs by the river's edge. Mindful walking can be so mind-calming."

Formal Walking Meditation

Any form of mindful walking will open up clear, fresh moments in your day and bring you into the present. If you would like to try a more formal practice, take some time outside or in a quiet room for the following meditation. (You may find it helpful to access a guided audio recording of this practice at www.nursingmindfully.com.)

Try This:
Formal Walking Meditation

Stand comfortably in a neutral position with your weight balanced and your spine in its natural position. Shift your weight to one leg, slowly lifting the other leg...starting to walk, relaxed but alert.

As you walk, notice each new movement and sensation as it passes into your awareness—lifting your foot, moving it, placing it down...just as a child discovers his feet and how to use them, exploring your body's movements as though for the first time, noticing also the sway of your arms.

If you lose focus, return your attention to the soles of your feet as they take turns touching the ground. When you notice your attention has wandered away, gently and patiently bring it back to the soles of your feet.

As your walking meditation comes to a close, set the intention to bring this feeling of calm into your next activity.

Journal Reflection:

Take a moment to reflect on your experience. What did you notice?

What, if anything, surprised you?

What sensations were you aware of during walking meditation?

Even in the commotion of a big city, you can walk with peace, happiness, and an inner smile. This is what it means to live fully in every moment of every day of your life.

—Thich Nhat Hanh

Noticing Tension and Embodied Emotions

Where do you experience your emotions? In your heart? In your mind? What about in your body?

You may seldom recognize the body as the arena where emotions play out. Yet if you are suddenly overcome with a rapid heart rate, red face, clenched jaw, trembling or shaking, you have no trouble interpreting the experience as anger, right?

Think about it. When you observe someone with slouching shoulders, a downturned mouth, and a torso that looks folded in on itself, you immediately sense that, whatever is happening, that person is not happy. Although you may often consider your thoughts and feelings as discreet and not observable by others, the body demonstrates what is being experienced. As a nurse, you see this play out every day when your intuition or "gut-feeling" tells you, based on your observations, what is going on, giving you valuable information about your patients. It's important to apply this same level of observation to what your own body is telling you.

Tense shoulders, neck, and back indicate stress and tension. Notice those moments in which you raise your shoulders and tighten your neck muscles throughout the day. Do you need a break? Is your body telling you that you need to relax? Probably.

Experiencing stomach upset, stomach ache, or butterflies in the tummy can suggest ongoing worry and anxiety. What is your gut trying to tell you?

Clenched fists, tightly crossed legs, or toes that dig into the ground signal anger or irritation. When you sense danger, you may unconsciously tighten your muscles and brace yourself. Moving slowly, feeling cold, or having a sluggish, droopy posture could point to being run-down, overworked, or depressed.

Becoming more aware of what your body is telling you is the first step toward acknowledging those feelings, which prevents them from becoming overwhelming.

Karen was a member of the Code Blue team. Although she worked in the ICU, whenever a code arrest was called anywhere in the hospital, she had to get there as quickly as possible. The stress of the call and Code Blue team responsibilities added to the stress of her shift, but every ICU nurse needed to take a turn. Going to so many codes frustrated Karen because it took time away from her other patients. She felt contempt for the codes, and whenever a code was called, she sighed and rolled her eyes. Once there, she pitched in and did her part, but the Code Blue responses took a lot out of her and she still needed to go back to her assignment in the ICU. Although she resented the situation, she felt guilty for feeling this way because she knew it was her job to take care of the sickest patients in the hospital.

Karen struggled with the difficult emotions these situations triggered, and she became reactive each time a code arrest was called. Unhelpful thoughts ran amok, increasing her feelings of stress and frustration. Perhaps you have found yourself in similar situations where, rather than being able to accept what was happening, you fought against it. With mindfulness, you can learn to identify and attend to difficult emotions as the body expresses them, exploring rather than suppressing them or acting out because of them. Relating to your emotions mindfully can help you feel more grounded and less reactive.

Try This:
Awareness of Emotions in the Body

Settle into a comfortable sitting position, upright yet relaxed, gently closing your eyes or softening your gaze.

Bring attention to your breathing, noticing the rhythm of your in-breath and out-breath.

(cont'd)

Bring to mind a difficult feeling or situation you have struggled with recently—something that provokes a strong emotion, such as anger or shame. This may feel uncomfortable, but stay with it if you can. You can always return your attention to your breath if the emotion becomes overwhelming.

Gently and kindly name your emotion. Is it anger, shame, sadness, grief? Perhaps more than one emotion is present.

Allow the emotion to be here, accepting it without trying to get rid of it or struggling against it.

Notice where you feel the emotion in your body. Perhaps there's a lump in your throat, heaviness in your chest, or tightness in your abdomen.

Bring a kind attention to this part of your body, allowing the sensations to be here, softening and opening to them…noticing whether the sensations change as you sit companionably with them.

Do you struggle to stay with them? Perhaps you find the emotion overwhelming —you replay an argument or relive feelings of rage, helplessness, or humiliation.

If feeling overwhelmed at any point, bring your attention back to your breath, allowing your focus to shift back and forth between the emotion and your breath.

When you find yourself thinking, "I wish I didn't feel this way" or "This feeling will never go away," return to a kind awareness of the sensations throughout your body…gradually bringing your attention to your breath and gently opening your eyes.

This practice helps you to stay present with difficult feelings throughout your day. When you open up to difficult emotions with a sense of kindness, you will feel more able to be with them and respond skillfully rather than reactively.

Journal Reflection:

How was this practice for you?

Which bodily sensations were you aware of?

Was this experience different from how you normally relate to difficult emotions?

It's like a mother, when the baby is crying, she picks up the baby and she holds the baby tenderly in her arms. Your pain, your anxiety, is your baby. You have to take care of it. You have to go back to yourself, to recognize the suffering in you, embrace the suffering, and you get a relief.

—Thich Nhat Hanh

Become aware of your body. If you frequently catch colds or other minor illnesses, reflect on your everyday stress and anxiety levels. What can you do to reduce the feelings of worry you experience every day? If not acknowledged, stress can elevate cortisol levels and weaken the immune system, making you more prone to illness.

Notice any changes in appetite or sleep cycles, such as insomnia or nightmares. Do you experience irregular menstrual cycles, acne breakouts, or allergy flare-ups? If so, these could be signs that your body and mind are rundown and in need of attention.

You feel better when you heed your body's messages. Remember to take time to indulge in a little self-care. Mindfulness will help you listen to your body and respond appropriately.

Practice Plan:

So far, you have been introduced to a variety of practices. If for any reason you can't try all of them, don't worry! Just do your best to make your daily practice your own in whatever way works for you. And most of all, make sure it fits in with your daily life and doesn't become one more obligation on your to-do list.

Before moving on to the next chapter, practice the body scan and walking meditation on alternate days for at least a week or two. If you can't make time or space for formal walking meditation, set the intention to walk mindfully during your shift. Again, focus on doing short body scans whenever the opportunity arises if you are not yet able to devote time to longer ones.

Keep up your informal practice by bringing mindful awareness to your daily activities and, throughout the day, bring your attention to sounds in your environment.

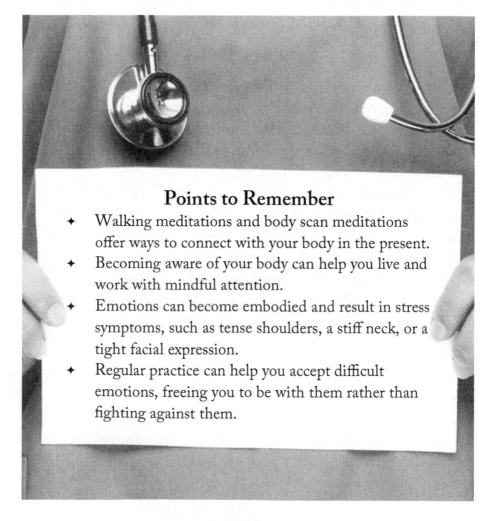

Points to Remember

+ Walking meditations and body scan meditations offer ways to connect with your body in the present.
+ Becoming aware of your body can help you live and work with mindful attention.
+ Emotions can become embodied and result in stress symptoms, such as tense shoulders, a stiff neck, or a tight facial expression.
+ Regular practice can help you accept difficult emotions, freeing you to be with them rather than fighting against them.

CHAPTER SEVEN

Preventing Injury the Mindful Way

Do not underestimate the power that comes to you from feeling the simple movements of your body throughout the day.

—Joseph Goldstein

Dee Burns loved night shift and working on the bariatric floor. She had an interest in surgery, and it made her feel good to help someone lead a more complete life without their extra pounds. Of course, lifting and moving these patients always presented the risk of injury, particularly back injury, but Dee was committed to taking care of herself when she lifted.

Special bariatric beds could mechanically lift an overweight patient, but these special beds were in short supply. Often, Dee had to move large patients on her own. One day, a large woman needed to be lifted up in bed.

As it happened, that day Dee was tired and stressed due to the number of patients on her assignment. With three coworkers helping, they lifted the patient to the head of the bed. Unfortunately, Dee forgot to bend her knees and use her legs as she lifted the patient. During the lift, Dee felt pain shoot down her leg, and she had a hard time standing up straight. Despite this, she continued her shift in pain, and finally, when the pain became unbearable, she told her supervisor. The facility doctor assessed Dee, and the MRI revealed she had a bulging disc in her back. Dee hadn't lifted her patient properly because she was too tired and stressed to pay proper attention. She was thinking about the number of total-lift patients she had under her care. In that one moment of distraction, she injured herself, and the injury required several weeks off work while she rehabilitated.

Do you experience muscular aches and pains? If so, it's not surprising. Musculoskeletal injuries are common among nurses like Dee because their work involves activities that can cause damage to, or wear and tear on, the body.

Consider This:

Have you ever found yourself skipping steps for safe lifting techniques when you felt rushed? Have you moved a patient by yourself instead of waiting for a coworker's help? Have you picked up an elderly patient and put him or her into their wheelchair, instead of using the mechanical lift? Do you look up from your charting only to realize your neck seems frozen in position?

The US Department of Labor's Bureau of Labor Statistics reports that nurses claimed nearly sixty-seven thousand cases of musculoskeletal disorders in 2013, and over thirty thousand of these resulted in a nurse losing at least one day of work.[19] The disorders ranged from back pain, sprains, and strains to tendinitis and carpal tunnel syndrome.

One study indicated an annual prevalence of these injuries in 40% to 50% of nurses, and stated that up to 80% sustain back injuries during their careers. Such injuries reduce work performance and increase absenteeism.[20]

Why Are Nurses Vulnerable to Injuries?

What is it about nursing that makes you more vulnerable to musculoskeletal injuries than people in other professions? The long hours of standing, bending, stretching, lifting, and reaching take their toll, especially when you repeat those movements every day.

Here are some common ways in which you might be at risk of injuring yourself:

- Standing for long hours during shifts or rounds
- Bending or standing at awkward angles for extended periods—for example, when bathing a patient or carrying out various procedures
- Heavy lifting, including supporting, lifting, or transferring patients and carrying heavy medical equipment
- Pushing wheelchairs and gurneys
- Reaching overhead to fetch heavy objects from shelves.

Ignoring Aches and Pains

The body, too, has its rights; and it will have them:
they cannot be trampled on without peril.

—*Guesses at Truth: by Two Brothers,*
by Julius Charles Hare and Augustus William Hare

Do you tune out that stiff upper back or that frozen shoulder? Beware! Your body is trying to tell you something.

Eileen Cameron loved working on the neurological unit, but the busyness of the unit and increased acuity of the patients were taking a toll on her body. In the beginning of her career, Eileen experienced pain only when she walked, and she reasoned that achy feet were part and parcel of nursing life, so she ignored her discomfort. Now, however, her condition descended into plantar fasciitis, and she could not walk the floor as a nurse must. Her doctor suggested time off, but that was impossible on her floor, so she applied for a manager position to reduce the time spent on her feet. This was a very difficult decision for her because she really enjoyed the patient care aspect of her work, but her health condition demanded that she make changes in her workload. Although she still worked on the same unit, her health problems limited the patient interaction that she enjoyed so much.

Over time, small aches or injuries like Eileen experienced may become chronic issues or cumulative trauma injuries. That niggling ache in your back may one day become full-blown, intense, debilitating back pain. The ache in your feet, knees, neck, or shoulder that once surfaced only at the end of long shifts perhaps now bothers you day and night. You may even be considering quitting your job or switching careers because your body just can't take it anymore. If this sounds like you, it is time to become mindful of what your body is telling you.

Mindfulness Prevents Injuries

Most injuries that occur in the course of nursing work result from poor ergonomics, bad posture, lack of awareness, or disregard for the body and its needs. Although overexertion, strenuous lifting, and bad posture are part of the problem, the bigger issue is the disconnect that exists between mind and body. You are most vulnerable to injuries when you are not aware of how you carry yourself or how you move. For instance, when you help a patient change sides, you might not notice that you are bending at an odd angle or straining your body. Becoming more mindful of your body—of how you lift, carry, and bend—helps to reduce these and other risks.

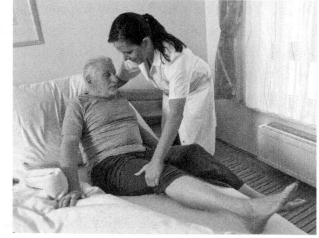

Become aware of how you feel as you move through your day. If you sense trouble in your body, don't ignore it. Does that shooting pain occur when you stand in a particular way to move a patient? If so, what can you do to change that?

Consider what supports must be put in place. Perhaps you can take a break, breathe deeply, or stretch as you move from one task to the next.

Mindful Posture

Attention to the human body brings healing and regeneration.
Through awareness of the body, we remember who we really are.

—Jack Kornfield

Good posture is crucial to orthopedic health. How you sit or stand plays a big role in preventing muscle injuries. Do you tend to slouch in your chair or hunch over your papers while making notes? When you are on your feet for too long, do you put more weight on one leg than the other? Do you move too quickly, without paying heed to your surroundings, constantly tripping over or banging into things?

You can prevent injuries by becoming more aware of how you move and by retraining your body to maintain good posture. As you go about your day, check whether your posture reflects your internal state. Let yourself move with care, honoring your body and inhabiting it with awareness.

If you regularly experience discomfort or tightness in a certain area, such as your lower back or shoulders, consider enrolling in a yoga or Pilates class, where you will learn exercises and stretches to relax and strengthen your body and prevent future injuries.

Belinda Kelly, a nurse on a cardiac floor, describes how she practices being mindful of her posture in the course of her workday. "Good posture was something I only heard about when I was growing

129

up. I had a habit of slouching, and my teachers would always tell me to straighten up. I hated to hear that!

"Since I started practicing mindfulness, I'm much more aware of how I'm sitting or standing. Sometimes at the nurses' station, I realize I'm slumping in my chair. Once I notice this, I'm able to make adjustments, but I have to set the intention to notice my posture throughout the day. Since I have been practicing poor posture for a lifetime, it is challenging to turn this around. When I'm changing linens for a patient who is in bed, I try to keep my back straight and my shoulders down. Likewise, I check my posture whenever I'm standing and waiting for a doctor to call back. Again, when waiting for the automatic blood pressure machine or for a patient to finish in the bathroom, I imagine a string on the top of my head, pulling me straight up into proper posture—shoulders down, muscles loose. Practicing this throughout my workday keeps me grounded and relaxed."

Becoming mindful of your posture is a great way to stay present. Set the intention to be mindful of your body as you go about your daily routine.

Try This:
Being in Your Body

Practice *being* in your body as you stand, sit, walk, or lie down, noticing the sensations as you turn and twist, when you bend and reach. What sensations are you aware of in your body right now? If you notice tension, allow it to dissolve on the out-breath.

Journal Reflection:

How mindful are you of your posture in the course of your workday? Are there any specific adjustments you need to make?

Mindful Lifting

The brain forgets much, but the lower back remembers everything.
—Robert Brault

Injuries happen when you lift heavy weights or move patients incorrectly. Take a moment to focus on your body before lifting and sustain that awareness until you finish, noticing which body parts or muscles you engage when you lift heavy objects. This awareness will give you greater control over how you use your body to lift and carry.

Be cautious. Use ergonomically smart techniques as well as machines to help you with weight bearing or lifting whenever you can. Do not lift a heavy patient on your own. Always ask for help.

Try This:
Mindful Lifting

Follow these basic rules:

Stand comfortably close to, and face the person (or object) that you intend to lift.

Squat with bent knees so your thighs take the main load, shifting the weight away from your lower back. Use your leg muscles rather than your back muscles to bear the weight of the person or object. You should feel the strain in your legs.

Keep a straight back and engage your abdominal muscles as you begin to lift.

Straighten your legs as you stand up, holding the person or object as close to your body as possible.

Chronic pain is a debilitating and limiting condition. Although many believe that such pain is a natural byproduct of aging, musculoskeletal injuries are not inevitable. By training yourself to be mindful of what you feel and how you move, you can reduce the risk of such injuries. When you are bending, lifting, or reaching, take a moment to notice what is going on in your body. Recognize even the subtlest sensations, making it a regular practice to tune in to how your body feels as you move around.

While being mindful of your body may not come naturally at first, with time it becomes a way of being, an important way of life.

Accidental Injuries and Illnesses

Hospitals and healthcare facilities can be dangerous environments, and nurses face danger every day from preventable accidents. Fortunately, mindfulness can help minimize these risks as you learn to pay attention and be aware of what is going on inside and around you.

We see the main cause of accidents is inattention and a lack of mindfulness about one's circumstances and surroundings.

—Marc Gomez

Skin Wounds: Needle-stick wounds can be hazardous due to the risk of communicable, blood-borne diseases. If carried incorrectly or mishandled, sharps may result in minor injuries or cuts that are more serious. Practice paying extra attention when using needles, scalpels, or other sharp instruments. Notice any distracting thoughts as you work with these instruments and return your attention to the task at hand.

Slips and Falls: Your work environment exposes you to hazards such as slips and falls. For example, because hospitals have high hygiene standards, it is necessary to disinfect floors regularly—which means workspaces and corridors may occasionally be slippery and increase your risk of tripping.

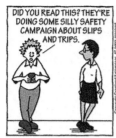 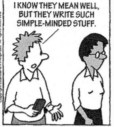 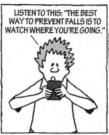 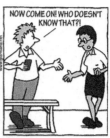

Falls can also occur when reaching for high shelves in storage rooms. If you have to climb a stepstool to retrieve extra linen or other equipment, be careful. As you walk, pay attention to your environment, noticing any hazards that could cause a fall, and wear shoes with good tread to reduce the risk of slipping.

Infections: Hospitals are the ultimate reservoir for infectious diseases. As you work, you could be exposed to anything from bacterial or viral infections to multi-resistant strains that cause severe illness. Potential exposure to infectious disease necessitates constant blood and body-fluid precautions, especially good handwashing. This can feel like a challenge when you are tired, stressed, or have underlying illnesses or injuries.

Let the ritual of washing your hands before and after treating each patient anchor you to the present. A mindless moment could cost a life!

Practice Plan:

Practice being mindful of your posture as you work, whether you are changing bed linen or lifting a patient. Continue to bring mindful awareness to everyday activities.

If you have been practicing the body scan or walking meditation for at least a week, you can now begin to alternate them with twenty minutes of sitting meditation on alternate days.

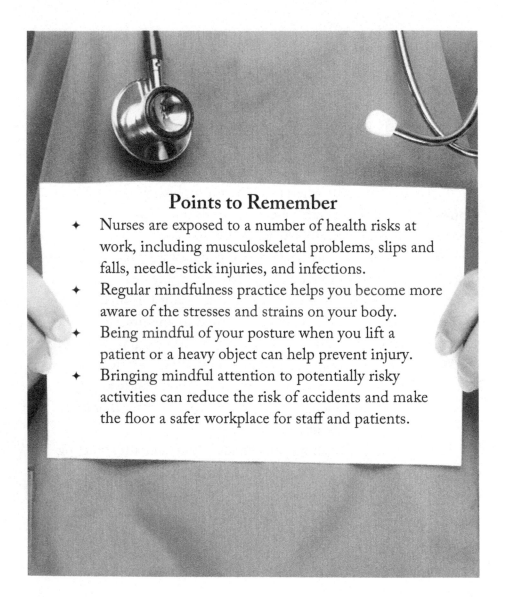

Points to Remember

✦ Nurses are exposed to a number of health risks at work, including musculoskeletal problems, slips and falls, needle-stick injuries, and infections.

✦ Regular mindfulness practice helps you become more aware of the stresses and strains on your body.

✦ Being mindful of your posture when you lift a patient or a heavy object can help prevent injury.

✦ Bringing mindful attention to potentially risky activities can reduce the risk of accidents and make the floor a safer workplace for staff and patients.

CHAPTER EIGHT

Coping Mindfully with Pain

When our pain is held by mindfulness, it loses some of its strength.
—Thich Nhat Hanh

Judy Loftus worked on an orthopedic floor, lifting patients with the help of anyone she could find among her coworkers. No matter how many years she worked on this unit, she was always careful of her back. One day, when lifting a heavyset man recovering from a hip replacement, Judy positioned the patient with the help of other staff but twisted her back in the process. The pain was immediate, and Judy collapsed to the floor.

The facility's doctor determined that Judy had torn a ligament in her knee and damaged her back at several vertebral levels. As a result, she was in rehab for months. Worker's compensation kept her going financially but soon pressured her to return to work. Eventually, she gave in and went back before she was ready.

Judy's pain was excruciating when she worked the floor. Often, she walked with a limp—and without a cane, although she really needed one. She could barely bend over to pick a tissue up off the floor, and when her back acted up, she would shut her eyes, grit her teeth, and try not to cry. Although Judy knew she wasn't ready to do this type of work, she felt she had no choice. It was either go back to work or lose her worker's compensation. She couldn't afford to lose the support, so she worked—despite her back and knee issues—and ignored the pain as best she could.

Unfortunately, Judy's story is not unique. Too many nurses have found themselves in a similar predicament: injured on the job but, due to financial constraints, unable to take enough time off to recover fully.

If you injure yourself, it is important to seek immediate attention, and prioritize your own self-care. Of course, the best thing is to prevent injury from occurring in the first place. That's where mindfulness comes in. If you are being mindful as you move, you are less likely to find yourself dealing with chronic aches and pains from continuous stress on your back, hands, and knees.

Do you begin your shifts by popping pain meds? Do you find yourself so overwhelmed by aches and pains that you have difficulty attending to your patients' needs? If so, you are not alone.

Nursing as a profession often involves physical injury. With injury comes pain. A 2011 study found that more than 90% of intensive care nurses experienced back pain at least once a month, and almost 22% had constant back pain. Another study found that more than half the nurses interviewed complained of chronic musculoskeletal pain, and for over a third, the pain was severe enough to require time off work. Of this group, 12% quit nursing, citing pain as a major contributor to their decision to leave.[21]

Consider This:

Do you tense up before any movement with the anticipation of pain? Have you ever considered falsely charting a patient's pain medication and then dispensing it to yourself? Have you ever had to fill out a worker's compensation form because of a work-related injury? How many times? How often have you said, "I'm getting too old for this? My back can't take it anymore"?

The good news is that you are not destined to a lifetime of pain and discomfort. Learning to deal mindfully with chronic pain may help you remain in your profession for many years to come.

What Is Pain?

What role does your mind play in your experience of physical pain? Everyone is different, and your reaction to pain may be different than Nurse Judy's or anyone else's.

The first step in experiencing pain is the sensation itself. This is the *sensory component* of pain. There are also the thoughts related to pain, such as, "How did it get so bad?" These thoughts make up the *cognitive component* of pain. Finally, there are emotions associated with pain and how it affects you. These feelings make up the *emotional component* of pain.

How do *you* react to pain?

Try This:
Exploring Difficult Sensations

Sit in a comfortable position and close your eyes.

Familiarize yourself with the sensations in your body, letting the aches and pains that have been in the background all day come into focus.

Zero in on the pain, investigating how the pain experience is for you.

Ask yourself: Is it a dull ache? A throbbing? A sensation of pinpricks? A stabbing pain? A pulsating sensation?

Notice any thoughts that are present, such as, "I hate that pain prevents me from working as much as I would like to."

Become aware of any emotions that are present. Perhaps you feel irritable, depressed, angry, or anxious.

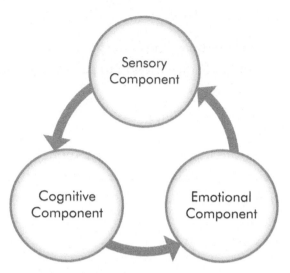

Figure 1. The Three Components of Pain

These sensory, cognitive, and emotional components come together to form your experience of pain. Each component feeds into the others and intensifies the experience. As your thoughts and nervous anticipation of feeling pain increase, the stronger the pain sensations will seem. The worse your sensations of pain become, the more negative your feelings and more intense your thoughts about it are likely to be.

Mindfulness and Pain

The normal response to pain is either to dwell on those negative thoughts and feelings, making the experience of pain worse, or to attempt to distract yourself from it with techniques such as guided imagery. Distraction can help when you are in acute pain and the symptoms are intense. On the other hand, with chronic pain, where the symptoms are mild to moderate, mindfulness is a better, more effective way to cope. As counterintuitive as this may sound, focusing attention on pain, or turning toward it, actually helps you to cope with it.

Two Kinds of Pain

Mindfulness distinguishes between two kinds of pain: primary and secondary. Primary pain is the immediate *sensation* of pain, whereas secondary pain is your *reaction* to the sensation. Secondary pain reactions often stem from feelings of anticipation and anxiety, which are fueled by thoughts such as, "This pain is the worst thing in the world," and "It will be crippling, and I will have to endure it for the rest of my life." These thoughts can exacerbate primary pain and add a "second arrow." The physical discomfort of pain is the first arrow and may be unavoidable, but the second arrow of counterproductive thoughts and negative emotions is entirely avoidable. Mindfulness helps you dodge the second arrow.

> *The attempt to escape from pain is what creates more pain.*
>
> —Gabor Mate

Earlier you read about Judy, who sustained an injury while lifting a patient. In the course of her rehabilitation, Judy learned how to work mindfully with pain. With practice, she was able to bring curiosity to the experience of pain when it was present, and as she did so, she noticed stretches of time when the pain was mild. Often, it would build in intensity and then over time subside. When the sensation was intense, she was able to shift her attention to a part of her body that wasn't in pain. She also noticed how the pain wasn't always present. Many times in the course of her day, she became aware of the absence of unpleasant sensations—she was pain-free.

Gradually, rather than bracing against pain, Judy was able to accept it. Instead of trying to tune out unpleasant sensations or becoming absorbed by them, she was more able to let them come and go. She also noticed that the more she thought about pain, the more she suffered. Over time, she began to realize how much she had been fighting against her experience and how the resistance actually made it worse. Judy gradually stopped resisting pain and instead was able to open up to her experience.

Although she still experienced pain at times, she began to realize these moments were transient; they would not last forever. As a result, her experience of pain was less debilitating, and she was able to face it and treat it with kindness. Eventually, she became more resilient to it and was able to get on with her life rather than being continually hijacked by unpleasant sensations.

Over time and with practice, mindfulness can change the way you respond to pain. When you are able to observe difficult sensations rather than judging them or reacting to them, you free yourself from secondary pain. For example, when you experience back pain, you may become aware of sensations of throbbing, tightness, heat, stabbing, radiating, pricking, or a dull ache. When you open up to these sensations, accepting them and breathing with them, eventually, the severity of pain diminishes to the extent that you will feel it less intensely or often not at all.

Try This:
Mindfulness of Difficult Sensations

Find a quiet place and settle into a comfortable position. Focus on your breathing, feeling your chest, abdomen, and shoulders rise and fall.

Once you feel relatively centered, slowly shift your focus to your pain zones, zeroing in on the general area of discomfort, paying attention to the sensations and trying to tease them apart. Is the pain throbbing or pulsing? Is it stabbing or radiating? Bring each sensation under a mental spotlight, welcoming it into your awareness.

(cont'd)

Now slowly turn your focus to the area where the pain is at its peak, observing it with as much attention as you can muster, noticing whether it changes as you observe it. Does it intensify? Is it milder?

If at any point the pain intensity becomes overwhelming, widen your awareness to other parts of your body. You can also gently move your awareness to your breathing if the pain becomes intense or overwhelming.

Return to exploring the pain sensations when you feel able to do so. If negative thoughts or feelings distract you, gently come back to the sensations, without judging them.

As you end the session, shift your focus back to your breathing, slowly returning your awareness to your surroundings.

Journal Reflection:

Take a moment now to reflect on your experience with this practice.

What did you notice when you focused on difficult sensations? Was this different from how you normally relate to pain?

When we feel pain, we should observe it as it is—pain.
—Chanmyay Sayadaw U. Janakabhivamsa

The good news is that you are not destined to a lifetime of pain and discomfort. Mindfulness can help reduce the intensity of pain by uncoupling the physical from the emotional and cognitive elements. Bringing mindful attention to sensations can help you break free of the difficult thoughts and feelings that intensify the experience of pain. By doing this, you build a higher pain threshold, and pain becomes a more manageable experience.

Practice Plan:

Continue alternating between the body scan, walking meditation, and sitting meditation every other day, and practice opening up to difficult sensations as you learned to do in this chapter. During your daily routine, continue bringing mindful awareness to your activities.

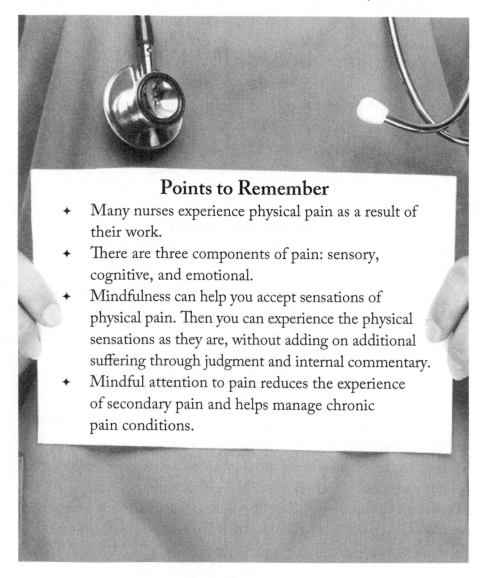

Points to Remember

+ Many nurses experience physical pain as a result of their work.
+ There are three components of pain: sensory, cognitive, and emotional.
+ Mindfulness can help you accept sensations of physical pain. Then you can experience the physical sensations as they are, without adding on additional suffering through judgment and internal commentary.
+ Mindful attention to pain reduces the experience of secondary pain and helps manage chronic pain conditions.

CHAPTER NINE

Coping with Stress the Mindful Way

We can easily manage if we will only take, each day, the burden appointed to it. But the load will be too heavy for us if we carry yesterday's burden over again today, and then add the burden of the morrow before we are required to bear it.

—John Newton

Kevin Larson always wanted to work in the emergency room. It was the primary reason he went into nursing, and he was over the moon when he was finally hired into the ER. It took him many hours of off-duty study to get up to speed with the tasks involved—assisting with intubation, spinal clearance, and inserting chest tubes emergently, to name but a few. Kevin soon realized, though, that working in the ER was not the ideal scenario he imagined it would be.

From the moment he arrived on the floor for his shift, Kevin was running. He took care of all kinds of patients—from those who were intoxicated or suffered minor lacerations to people with Alzheimer's who couldn't communicate their needs. Some patients were admitted to the floor, and as the assigned nurse, Kevin would have to escort them to their rooms. When he returned to the ER, his rooms were full again, and he had to start all over, taking histories, gathering vitals, and assessing the primary cause of injury or illness. As Kevin went through these steps with every new patient, he felt stressed trying to keep up with it all. Everyone in the ER wanted to be seen immediately, and in one night he might assist twenty to thirty patients over his twelve-hour shift. When he didn't get to them fast enough, they would demand his attention by ringing their bells.

From the outset, Kevin wanted to work directly with trauma patients, but it wasn't easy to make this happen. Although everyone wants to be on the trauma team, doctors, interns, and more experienced nurses normally get the privilege of working with the most severely ill or injured. Most of the time, Kevin was left outside the trauma room with no help while the team worked inside.

The ER quickly lost its luster for Kevin, falling far short of his expectations. He was stressed-out and disillusioned. Eventually, it got so bad that he developed an ulcer. His hair began to fall out, and he was always fatigued from running around the unit. He considered moving to a different department but had already spent time on a med-surg floor, and he didn't like that either. Kevin decided he had to face facts: nursing was apparently not for him. He was ready to quit as soon as he found a less stressful job.

A survey of ten thousand nurses conducted by the Royal College of Nursing showed that almost two-thirds had considered quitting their job because of stress.[22] When you think about the demanding schedule, long shifts, unpredictable hours, working under pressure, and caring for the seriously ill and dying, is this statistic surprising?

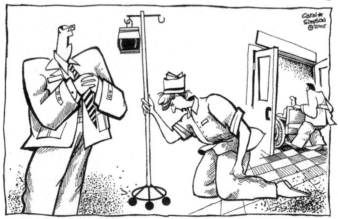

"You're in a hospital, Nurse Hill. If you collapse from exhaustion, the emergency room is just down the hall."

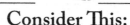

Consider This:

Has nursing lost its luster for you? Do you find yourself going through the online job boards on your days off? Following a stretch of days off, do you feel depressed the night before you have to return to work? Are your sleep patterns in disarray? Do you suffer from regular stomach upset? Do you find yourself doubting your nursing abilities?

Nurses work in the foxhole of the healthcare battlefield. Their work is emotionally grueling and physically draining. Routine stressors are bad enough, but factor in the bad days where mistakes are made, coworkers are unhelpful, patients die, or the workload is unsafe, and what *is* surprising is that 38% of those nurses have *not* considered quitting the profession!

Stress is nearly impossible to avoid. You may feel it while driving, working, interacting with your loved ones, or waiting in line at the local pharmacy. Stress dramatically reduces vitality and zest for life, impacting health, relationships, mental acumen, and spiritual wholeness. In the end, it can make each day feel like a chore.

How Stressed Are You?

How would you rate your stress level? Use The Nursing Stress Scale below to find out. This scale lists thirty-four situations that commonly occur on a hospital unit and cause stress for nurses in the course of their work. Four response categories are provided for each situation: Never (0), Occasionally (1), Frequently (2), Very frequently (3). Indicate by means of a checkmark (√) how often on your present unit you have found each situation to be stressful.

Item	Never (0)	Occasionally (1)	Frequently (2)	Very frequently (3)
Factor One: Workload				
Breakdown of the computer				
Unpredictable staffing and scheduling				
Too many non-nursing tasks required, such as clerical work				
Not enough time to provide emotional support to a patient				
Not enough time to complete all of my nursing tasks				
Not enough staff to adequately cover the unit				
Factor Two: Death and Dying				
Performing procedures that patients experience as painful				
Feeling helpless in the case of a patient who fails to improve				
Listening or talking to a patient about his/her approaching death				
The death of a patient				
The death of a patient with whom you developed a close relationship				
Physician not being present when a patient dies				
Watching a patient suffer				
Factor Three: Inadequate Preparation				
Feeling inadequately prepared to help with the emotional needs of a patient's family				
Being asked a question by a patient for which I do not have a satisfactory answer				
Feeling inadequately prepared to help with the emotional needs of a patient				
Factor Four: Lack of Staff Support				
Lack of an opportunity to talk openly with other unit personnel about problems on the unit				
Lack of an opportunity to share experiences and feelings with other personnel on the unit				
Lack of an opportunity to express to other personnel on the unit my negative feelings toward patients				

Item	Never (0)	Occasionally (1)	Frequently (2)	Very frequently (3)
Factor Five: Uncertainty Concerning Treatment				
Inadequate information from a physician regarding the medical condition of a patient				
A physician ordering what appears to be inappropriate treatment for a patient				
A physician not being present in a medical emergency				
Not knowing what a patient or a patient's family ought to be told about the patient's medical condition and its treatment				
Uncertainty regarding the operation and functioning of specialized equipment				
Factor Six: Conflict with Physicians				
Criticism by a physician				
Conflict with a physician				
Fear of making a mistake in treating a patient				
Disagreement concerning the treatment of a patient				
Making a decision concerning a patient when the physician is unavailable				
Factor Seven: Conflict with Other Nurses				
Conflict with a supervisor				
Floating to other units that are short-staffed				
Difficulty in working with a particular nurses (or nurses) outside the unit				
Criticism by a supervisor				
Difficulty in working with a particular nurse (or nurses) on the unit				

With permission of James G. Anderson, PhD, Purdue University[23]

The total score results can range from 0 to 102, and the higher your score, the greater your stress level. Stress is categorized as low with a score from 0 to 34; moderate with a score from 35 to 68; or high with a score from 69 to 102.

Journal Reflection:

Following completion of the scale, take some time to reflect on work situations that you experience as stressful. Is any one of the seven sub-areas of the scale particularly stressful for you? If your score was at the high end of the scale, reflect for a moment on anything you have learned. Did anything surprise you? Is it within your power to change any of the situations you identified as stressful?

Understanding Stress

Stress is to the human condition what tension is to the violin string: too little and the music is dull and raspy; too much and the music is shrill or the string snaps. Stress can be the kiss of death or the spice of life.

—*The Stress Solution*, by Lyle H. Miller,
Alma Dell Smith, and Larry Rothstein

In your training as a nurse, you learned about the physiology of stress. When a person perceives something as a threat, the brain sends signals to the nervous systems. Once that happens, the endocrine system shifts into overdrive, secreting the stress hormones epinephrine and cortisol. The body directs attention to dealing with the threat at hand and reacts with symptoms such as sweating, racing pulse, and shaking. Once the threat is gone, the system reverts to normal function.

This fight-or-flight response evolved for a specific purpose: to release quick energy into the bloodstream. It is the natural, lifesaving, game-changing response to an emergency. If a gunman suddenly entered the emergency room where you were working, then this response would mobilize you to either flee or fight the danger. Once security had him in handcuffs and everyone was safe, your body would gradually return to normal homeostasis.

In today's fast-paced, ultracompetitive world, stressors do not typically come in the form of immediate danger that you can choose to flee or fight. Instead, modern stressors are things like work-related deadlines, strained relationships, health issues, and financial setbacks. Add to that short staffing and poor working conditions. No task force will swoop in to the rescue, so these threats do not disappear quickly. They are pervasive. Instead of returning to normal homeostasis, your body continues to pump out cortisol.

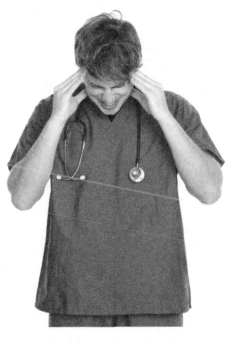

This unremitting undercurrent of tension and the ongoing low-level, fight-or-flight state leaves your body constantly stressed and wreaks havoc on your nervous system, throwing your hormonal balance into disarray. Your pulse may periodically race, you may frequently break into a sweat, and your sleep and appetite may be repeatedly disrupted.

Stress Reaction versus Stress Response

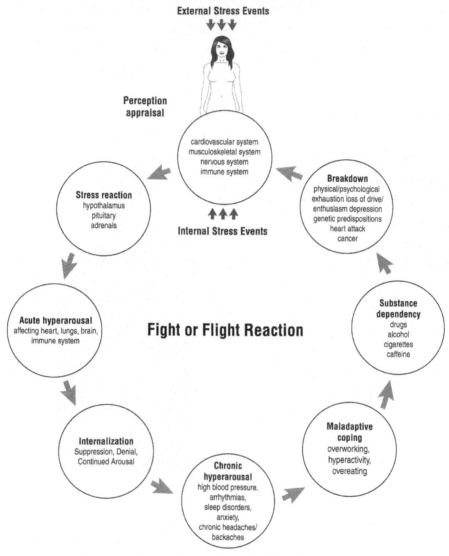

Figure 2.[24] The Fight-or-Flight Reaction

In a stress reaction, an external stressor acts as the trigger. It can happen at any time and can be anything from dealing with a difficult patient to running late on your rounds. Your mind appraises the stimulus and quickly forms opinions about it, such as "The patient is unhappy with me. I must be a terrible nurse." The mental reaction is a critical stage in your response because your opinions, or perceptions, of the trigger determine whether or not your body will have a stress reaction to it.

Your negative assessment of the situation triggers a reaction of acute hyperarousal in your body. The physical symptoms that accompany stress are based on fight-or-flight reactivity. Blood flow diverts to your limbs to prepare your body to fight or flee. Blood pressure rises, your pulse speeds up, your mouth goes dry, and you begin to sweat.

At this point, behavioral reactions kick in. For instance, you avoid the patient or react defensively or with hostility. Then you may feel guilty, your patient may become more hostile, and patient care may suffer as a result. Perhaps you try to minimize the stress by internalizing it—denying it or "putting on a happy face." This happens often with long-term stressors—such as poor working conditions, or patients who are constantly demanding. While you may be able to push the stressor further from your mind—or comfort yourself later with a snack or a stiff drink— you can't avoid the effects over the long term.

Eventually, you slip into dysregulation, with your body no longer in acute but in chronic hyperarousal, which causes problems with your cardiovascular, musculoskeletal, nervous, and immune systems. To compound the problem, your reaction to the stressor may lead you into maladaptive coping behaviors, such as working or eating too much and substance dependency (drugs, alcohol, cigarettes, caffeine).

This stress reaction is a vicious circle in which your reaction at any point in the cycle triggers additional stress reactions with which your body and mind must cope. All these stressors then lead to physical and psychological breakdowns. Yet, you may be unaware you are stressed until you reach the point of burnout. In an attempt to be more productive, you might go through day after day of frenzied activity, sweeping negative emotions under the carpet and carrying around pent-up stress.

Stress Reaction versus Stress Response

Be present as the watcher of your mind, of your thoughts and emotions as well as your reactions in various situations. Be at least as interested in your reactions as in the situation or person that causes you to react.

—Eckhart Tolle

Mindfulness turns things around by heightening awareness of your thoughts, feelings, and reactions. This helps you to become centered at will and to break the cycle and *respond,* rather than *react,* to the situation.

Imagine that you have had a disagreement with a colleague. Perhaps you become physically tense. Feelings of hostility and sadness about a relationship-gone-sour emerge. Later, at home, you relive the disagreement through a "postmortem" on what was said and done. Lost in your narrative of what occurred, resentment festers and causes unpleasant feelings, and possibly further friction.

Stress is a cycle of three components: physical tension, painful emotions, and rumination. For instance, your disagreement might have resulted in physical tension such as hunched shoulders, clenched fists, or neck pain. Along with this came feelings of hostility, often related to fear and anxiety. What might the argument mean for your friendship or working relationship? Rumination is the final step in the cycle. When you get home, you brood on your experience, going over it again and again.

When you become stressed, you get caught in this cycle. Rather than noticing physical sensations, feelings, and thoughts triggered during the disagreement, you get lost in the story of what happened. Rumination, the final part of the stress cycle, can be particularly destructive because it continues to ramp up your physical and emotional stress long after the incident is over.

Fortunately, mindfulness can help break the cycle of stress, and with practice, you can notice sensations, feelings, and unhelpful ruminations as they arise, rather than getting lost in them. Eventually, this helps you unhook from the storyline and frees you from reactivity.

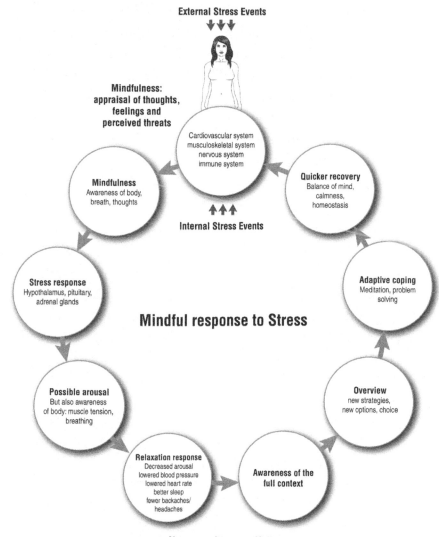

Figure 3. [24] Responding Mindfully to Stress

When you are mindful, you take stock of your feelings and thoughts in their full context and assess if the threat is real or merely *perceived*. Rather than being caught in the reactive cycle, you are able to see *new options* that you didn't think of previously. Then, rather than over-eating, over-working, or drinking, you can respond with *adaptive coping* skills. For example, you calm yourself with mindful breathing or reach out to a friend for support. You reverse the physiological stress response, and your body and mind return to a balanced state. With practice, this mindful response becomes more ingrained, and you can access it readily in challenging situations.

The key to becoming less reactive and more responsive to stress lies in the awareness that *you have a choice*. You are not the helpless victim of your circumstances. Clearly, you have the power to respond to stressful situations more skillfully.

Try This:
Respond Mindfully to Stress

When you encounter a challenging situation, take a mindful pause and become centered, feeling your feet touching the floor.

Notice what is going on in your body and mind.

Is your heart thumping? Has your breathing quickened?

Notice any thoughts such as, "This patient could get me fired."

Name any feelings that are present, such as anger or fear.

As you take a breath, observe the patient's attitude without personalizing it.

If you notice that you have become lost in thought, silently say the word "thinking." Return your attention to your breath, your body, or to what you are doing.

(cont'd)

This practice helps you to *respond* rather than *react* to the situation. Although you may still feel upset, you will be less embroiled in the stress and better able to let it go so it no longer affects the rest of your day.

As you unhook from the story, in time, you may begin to see the situation from a wider perspective. Maybe a different thought arises: "This patient must be really ill and uncomfortable, and that's why he is being so abrupt and hostile."

Between stimulus and response, there is a space. In that space is our power to choose our response. In our response lies our growth and our freedom.

—Viktor Frankl

Recognize Stress in Your Body

Do not wait until your body is flooded with stress hormones before you practice mindfulness. By then, it is often too late! Instead, practice being mindful when things are going smoothly and during the early stages of stress. The more you practice, the easier it becomes to zero in on the early warning signs while they are being triggered. As you will discover, this helps to interrupt the stress reaction and prevents it escalating.

With the constant demands of today's healthcare environment, adrenaline may be the only thing that gets you through your day. However, stress reactions need not be all that steers you through life. After all, there is another, healthier way—one more beneficial to your life and your career.

Observe yourself mindfully. Free yourself from unhelpful ruminating thoughts and choose to respond differently to stress. You *can* break the negative cycle. Furthermore, you can now use the time and energy you save for positive interactions with yourself, your patients, and your loved ones. Begin responding to the stress in your life, rather than reacting to it!

Practice Plan:

This week, when you encounter potentially stressful situations, use the three-step breathing space to cope. Continue practicing either the body scan, sitting meditation, or walking meditation on alternate days. Reflect on your experience in your journal.

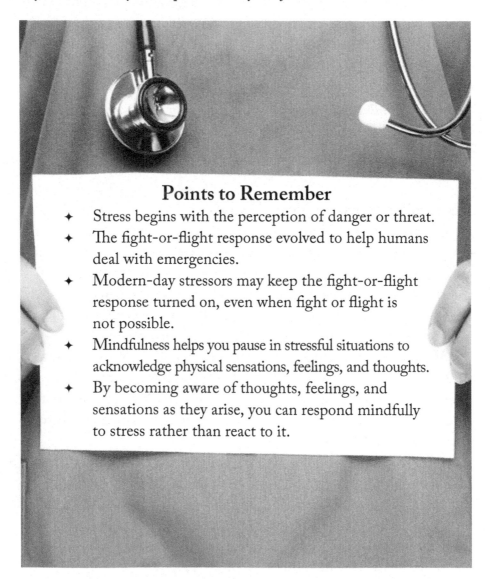

Points to Remember

✦ Stress begins with the perception of danger or threat.
✦ The fight-or-flight response evolved to help humans deal with emergencies.
✦ Modern-day stressors may keep the fight-or-flight response turned on, even when fight or flight is not possible.
✦ Mindfulness helps you pause in stressful situations to acknowledge physical sensations, feelings, and thoughts.
✦ By becoming aware of thoughts, feelings, and sensations as they arise, you can respond mindfully to stress rather than react to it.

CHAPTER TEN
Mindful Movement

A meditation that involves moving ... can shift us from one mental mode to another. Tai chi, chi gung, and hatha yoga are all moving meditations.

—Jon Kabat-Zinn

As a new nurse working in the burn unit at her local hospital, Ellen Hanley was drawn to natural, holistic ways to cope with the stress in her life. When she was in college, she had attended a local yoga class with a friend. She found it liberating as it took her mind off her schoolwork. For that hour, nothing else existed as she focused on the sensations in her body. Much as Ellen enjoyed yoga, she didn't do it regularly after college. Her life was busy with other things.

When she began work on the burn unit, Ellen found herself inundated with patients who had lost most of their skin. Bandages needed to be changed daily—often multiple times— and the narcotics she gave didn't always alleviate the pain. After a brutal and emotional shift on the floor, Ellen's shoulders would be tight and her head would throb. She couldn't stop thinking about the events that occurred during her shift—such as the child with third-degree burns over 75% of his body. When Ellen felt on the verge of emotional collapse, the friend who had encouraged her to try yoga in the first place suggested she try it again.

But Ellen was reluctant. "Who has time for stretching and silly postures?" she thought. Besides, it would take more than that to help her cope with the emotional trauma she felt every day. But her friend persisted, and Ellen finally gave in. To her surprise, the obsessive thoughts she had about work evaporated once she focused on moving and stretching her body. As before, in that hour, she found great relief as she opened herself up to relaxation. Initially, Ellen thought she didn't have time or energy for yoga. Now, she can't do without it.

Consider This:

Do you feel so emotionally and/or physically drained after work that all you want to do is sleep? Does your back hurt so much when you crawl into bed that you need to place pillows under your legs just to get comfortable? Are you convinced that you can't possibly fit an exercise program, or meditation time, into your busy lifestyle?

Given the hazards of the nursing profession, it is important to do all that you can to stay fit and healthy in both mind and body. By protecting yourself from injury, you can function at your best, deliver the required level of care, and continue working in your chosen profession. The National Health System (NHS) in the United Kingdom is acutely aware of the dangers posed by occupational back injuries and advocates measures to help nurses reduce the chance of injury and alleviate symptoms of existing injuries. One activity the NHS specifically advocates is yoga.[25]

Yoga postures are often used as the foundation for movement practice in mindfulness training. Like yoga, tai chi and chi gung are also mindful movement practices that use slow, smooth body movements combining present-centered awareness and concentration.

Often called "Chinese yoga," chi gung uses breathing techniques, gentle movement, and meditation to improve health and healing. It can include static, standing, or fluid exercises. Tai chi is a form of chi gung in a choreographed series of postures that can range from a few to over a hundred. Although the movements of tai chi and chi gung are similar, chi gung movements are usually easier, making it accessible to practically anyone wanting to learn an authentic mind-body practice.

Whatever the form, mindful movement practice is more of an exercise of the mind than of the body. The tai chi saying, "We use the body, but we practice the mind," applies from the beginning of the practice when you set the intention to relinquish the goal of physical achievement for the intention of cultivating awareness of mind and body.

A mindful approach to movement helps to lower stress, increase energy, improve concentration, raise body awareness, promote relaxation, and decrease the incidence of injury. Science has verified that yoga, chi gung, and tai chi improve balance and flexibility while increasing harmony of mind, body, and spirit.

Mindful movement sharpens the quality of awareness, enabling you to become mindful as you move. It is not just an exercise regimen or a keep-fit program—it is meditation in action. Mindful movement can become a way of life that will help you live fully in the present.

As you practice, you learn to tune in to your body and consciously *be* in it, noticing your breathing and the sensations that arise as you move. This focus quiets the mind, allowing body and mind to gradually settle into a relaxed and meditative state.

Mindful movement helps you build awareness of your body. In the rush of your daily routine, you may forget to pay full attention to your bodily sensations. For instance, you might not notice when you clench your jaw or tense your neck and shoulder muscles. Regular practice helps you develop a stronger relationship between your body and mind, making you aware of what your body is doing and feeling. Eventually, this allows you to spot tension before it translates into a strain, ache, or headache. Once you acknowledge what's present in your body, you can respond appropriately. For instance, if you notice that your breathing is ragged, you can ease up and pace yourself as you move through your day.

Paying attention to and staying with finer and finer sensations within the body is one of the surest ways to steady the wandering mind.
—Ravi Ravindra

Investigate your Limits

By working with relatively slow, careful movements such as yoga, tai chi, or chi gung sequences, and tuning in to your physical sensations as you move, you can explore and become familiar with your body's limits or "edges." Your "edge" is the limit of what is comfortable for you, the point where you feel you are being challenged to the max by intense sensations. As you stretch and balance throughout the sequence, the place where your comfort begins to be challenged will reveal itself. You may actually injure yourself if you go beyond this point. What matters most is that you listen to your body and its messages.

Becoming aware of this limit, exploring it with sensitivity, and moving with its subtle shifts but without forcing your way through it, is called "playing the edge." Through mindful movement, you will gradually begin to notice your habit of dealing with your edge when you encounter it. You can learn a lot about yourself from your pattern of reacting. For example, do you have a tendency to strive too hard and slam your way through difficult experiences or pull back too quickly to avoid discomfort? Both extremes have their downside. Through mindful movement, you may gradually discover a new way to handle difficulty. Rather than pushing yourself too far or giving up too easily, when you pay mindful attention, you will be able to choose wisely how far to go with a stretch and how long to hold it.

What is required of us is that we love the difficult and learn to deal with it.
In the difficult are the friendly forces, the hands that work on us.
—Rainer Maria Rilke

In the same way, you can begin to explore how you relate to emotional pain and other edges in your life. We often stay away from both our physical and mental edges by keeping within a familiar but limited comfort zone. By intentionally bringing your body to its different edges and holding it there, gently easing in toward more openness, you can learn new and kinder ways of being with difficult emotions and experiences in your life. You will discover that your limits are not fixed, but can expand and change. This can be very freeing.

Mindful Movement: Sitting Stretches

You can now try out a mindful movement practice through the following sequence of poses. The aim of this practice is to tune in to the unfolding sensations in your body, noticing your limits or edges. As you practice, allow the eight foundational attitudes of mindfulness to guide you: beginner's mind, patience, non-judging, non-striving, trust, self-compassion, letting go, and acceptance.

Notice any judgments or thoughts pushing you toward extending further than feels comfortable and safe for your body. When this happens, gently return your awareness to your breath and sensations. Notice if any stretches make you feel sad, irritated, angry, or fearful. If you change your breathing, how does that affect the feeling?

Depending on the time you have available, you can do the entire sequence or, alternatively, individual poses. If you are a beginner, review all of the illustrations before you start the practice so as to learn the sequence. Knowing the order of the poses will add to the flow of your session.

Rhythmically repeat each movement three or four times, if that feels comfortable for you, before moving to the next pose. As with any exercise, you can loosen up and warm up before beginning by gently swinging your limbs or slowly rotating your joints. Move within and between poses gradually. Start by holding the pose for a short length of time, gradually increasing the time as your practice improves.

If you have any injuries or medical concerns, be sure to discuss them with your doctor in advance. Seek out the guidance of a yoga instructor who can help you modify or avoid various poses as needed.

The breath is considered the link between the mind and the body and should take center stage in your awareness as you practice mindful movement. When you move through a pose, the movement and your breath will become naturally coordinated because movement is associated with in-breaths and out-breaths, as you breathe in and out through your nose. The mind and body experience harmony when breathing is coordinated with movement. In the stretches that follow, use your breath as your guide. If your breath is ragged or if holding the pose doesn't feel good, these are signals for you to ease up and come out of the pose.

To coordinate breath with movement, you can follow these general guidelines:

- Breathe in when extending.
- Breathe out when contracting.
- Breathe in when rising.
- Breathe out when lowering.
- Breathe out when going into a twist.
- Breathe in coming out of a twist.

Try This:
Seated Poses

Throughout this sitting practice, notice the muscles in the body tensing and relaxing, and observe what is happening with the breath. Remember that your intention is simply to explore what is present in your body and mind rather than create anything special.

Pose 1: Seated Forward Fold

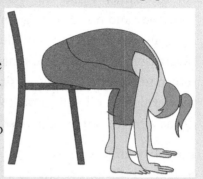

Find a comfortable seat on a chair, placing your feet flat on the floor, hip-width apart. With your spine long and shoulders back, slowly move your body forward so your back is away from the chair. Reaching your arms overhead, begin to fold forward, bending at the hip (not the waist) and allowing your arms to follow. Breathe in and out of the pose, mindfully exploring your edge, noticing any unnecessary clenching in the jaw, eyes, or abdomen. Gently lifting your arms as you return to an upright seat. Repeat.

Pose 2: Seated Twist

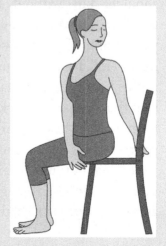

With your feet on the floor in front of you, twist your torso to the left, reaching your left hand toward the back of the chair and your right hand across your body toward the outside of your left leg. At the point where you feel you have gone as far as you comfortably can, pause and breathe deeply. Repeat the pose, this time on your right side. Do several repetitions.

(cont'd)

Pose 3: Seated Eagle

Sitting comfortably, cross your left leg over your right leg. Bring your arms up, crossing the left underneath the right. Intertwine your arms, reaching your palms back around until they touch. Move up close to the edge of your comfort zone. What do you notice in your body and mind? Using your breath, bring awareness to your shoulders, taking several breaths and releasing. Gently return to a normal sitting position. Hug your arms around your torso to relax out of the stretch. Repeat the pose on the opposite side.

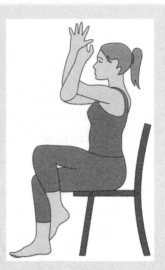

Pose 4: Seated Neck Rolls

Seat yourself on a chair. With your spine long and the crown of your head reaching toward the sky, drop your chin toward your chest. Use your breath to bring your head up and toward the left, tilting your left ear over your left shoulder but without bringing them together. Breathe here, gently exploring your limit, then allow your chin to slowly roll back to your chest. If you notice your attention has wandered off into thinking, come back to exploring sensations. Use the breath to move your head up and over the right shoulder, again taking your ear over your shoulder, but not bringing them together, stretching but not straining. Repeat on each side an equal number of times, then gently take your chin back to your chest, and slowly lift your head back up to a neutral position.

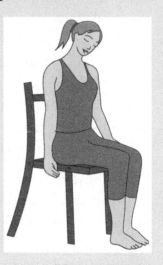

(cont'd)

Standing Poses

Pose 5: Mountain Pose

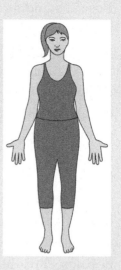

Stand with your feet a little ways apart—left foot positioned below the left hip, right foot below the right hip. Feel both feet underneath you, keeping your knees soft, or very slightly bent. Extend the crown of your head toward the sky, allowing your shoulders to slide away from your ears to rest on the back of the body. Bring awareness to your back, inhaling and exhaling several times. Gradually, become aware of your feet in contact with the earth and the sense of being grounded and supported. Notice any feelings that are present.

Pose 6: Plank

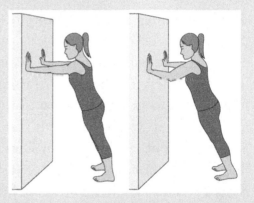

Place your palms in front of you on a wall—at shoulder height and shoulder-distance apart—standing an arm's length away. Spread your fingers, pressing into the wall as though you were holding it away from you. Keeping your elbows close to your body, lean into the wall as though moving into a low pushup. Using your breath as your guide, move in and out from one part of the pose to the other. Notice what happens in your body when you breathe in and what happens when you breathe out. Hold at the wall for several seconds before slowly pushing away. Repeat the exercise, increasing the number of repetitions as your body becomes accustomed.

(cont'd)

Pose 7: Standing Modified

Standing upright in the mountain pose, bring your palms to your lower back (at your waistline). Reach your elbows behind you as though they could touch. Gently lean back into your palms, dropping your head back and relaxing your neck. Explore your edge by carefully tuning into your physical sensations, listening to your body, and honoring its limits. Gradually lift back up through your chest into an upright position, breathing into and out of the pose.

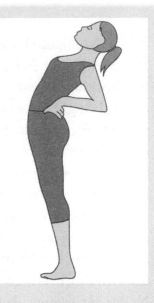

Pose 8: Standing Knees to Chest

Stand with your feet a little ways apart, assuming the mountain pose. Bring your awareness to the right side of the body, placing your weight on your right foot. If you comfortably can, slowly lift your left leg to your chest, hugging your arms around it. Hold for several seconds. Noticing any thoughts or emotions that arise, as well as what is happening in your body, breathing into any areas of discomfort. Slowly release the left leg back to the floor, bringing your right leg up to the chest. Repeat several times on each side.

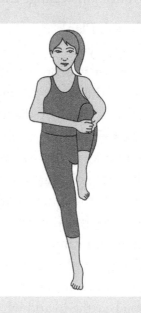

(cont'd)

Pose 9: Tree

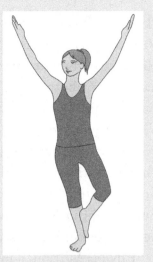

Stand with your feet a little ways apart, assuming the mountain pose. Bring your weight onto your left leg. At whatever height your body allows, place your right foot on the inside of your left leg, anywhere on the leg except directly on the knee. If you are unaccustomed to balancing on one leg, then place your right leg closer to the ground or leave your toes touching the floor. You can keep your arms at your side or lift them. Hold for several seconds, paying attention to the shifting sensations, gently playing with your edge of comfort. Repeat on the left side, and then return to the mountain pose.

To end this sequence of postures, remain in mountain pose for some moments. Slowly scan your body, noticing any change in sensations following these gentle stretches. Breathe with awareness of the whole body.

Journal Reflection:

What did you notice during this practice?

Were you aware of any particular sensations?

Did you notice unpleasant sensations associated with particular stretches?

Were you able to open to the experience of unpleasantness, and breathe into those sensations?

Was there a tendency to push past your limits or to work with them kindly and sensitively?

Were you judging your body on the basis of what you can or cannot do?

Were you aware of any emotions?

How did you feel immediately after the practice?

Mindful Movement at Work

With practice, you can bring the awareness cultivated during mindful movement into your daily life. As a result, you will find that you can better give full attention to your breathing, to what you are doing, and to how you are moving throughout your day. Whether you are giving out medication, charting, setting up a drip, moving a patient, going on ward rounds, or engaging in other activities, you will notice more how your body feels. When you notice tension in your neck or shoulder muscles or feel that your breathing is shallow, you can take gentle action to remedy the trouble before it escalates.

Edwina Wilson, a nursing assistant on a busy ICU step-down unit, describes how she uses every opportunity to integrate mindful movement into her day. "Every morning I do some gentle stretching before my shift starts. This helps calm my mind and prepare my body for the day ahead. My shift goes more smoothly and I have more energy, which helps me be more productive. Whenever I have a spare moment in my day, I stop and stretch. When I use the bathroom, I take a moment to do a yoga pose. When my coworkers are outside having a smoke break, I join them but instead of smoking, I stretch. Since I've been doing this, I notice my thoughts are less stressed and my body doesn't ache so much when I come home after my shift."

Like Edwina, you can incorporate mindful movement into your workday to keep stress at bay. Short moments of practice can provide a wealth of immediate physical and emotional benefits: pain relief, improved energy and concentration, and reduced stress and tension.

Do you feel that your schedule and the demands of work leave no time for mindful movement? In the course of your workday, do you tend to opt for nicotine, unhealthy snacks, or caffeine for energy boosts, even though you know these quick fixes are short-lived?

If you need something to energize your body and calm your mind during the workday, substitute positive practices that will protect you from stress, exhaustion, depression, injury, and pain. Mindful movement allows you to press your body's "reset button" and helps you to let go of tension—physical and mental—and breathe properly again.

Remember to take a minute or two to do some mindful stretches during coffee or bathroom breaks in the course of your shift. If you make this a habit, your body and mind will reap the benefits!

Practice Plan:

Take a pause from reading this book before moving on to the third section. Doing so will give you time and space to integrate the practices you have learned so far. Over the course of the next few weeks, keep up your formal daily practice, exploring different combinations of mindful movement, sitting meditation, and walking meditation.

Continue to bring mindful awareness to your daily activities. Finally, resume reading the book when you have integrated these practices into your daily routine.

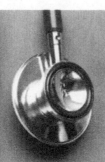
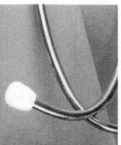

Points to Remember

+ The aim of mindful movement practice is to allow you to tune in to your body, breath, sensations, thoughts, and emotions as you move in a way that brings harmony and balance.
+ Through mindful movement, you become familiar with your limits or "edges" of resistance and how you deal with them.
+ It is important to listen to your body during mindful movement practice, and respect, rather than push through, its limitations.
+ Mindful movement is a practice that works anywhere. You can even practice during breaks at work to keep stress and back pain at bay.

PART III
COMPASSION—THE ESSENCE OF MINDFULNESS

It is compassion that removes the heavy bar, opens the door to freedom, makes the narrow heart as wide as the world.

—Nyanaponika Thera

CHAPTER ELEVEN

Understanding Compassion

If you want to be happy, practice compassion.
—Dalai Lama

Practicing meditation and developing mindfulness leads to a greater awareness of the moment, an ability to focus with clarity, and a less egocentric view of the world. Mindfulness leads to a deeper understanding of your own experience and a keener sense of what others are feeling.

Recent research strongly suggests a connection between mindfulness and compassion. By fostering focus and emotional control, mindfulness not only enables greater awareness of another person's experience but also leads to more compassionate action.

Mary Kennedy, a nurse and manager for several years, was always more than willing to try any means to help her patients, and didn't feel that traditional medicine had all the answers. With some work, she became a certified holistic nurse and went into private practice with two of her school friends.

The patients Mary saw had usually reached their limits with traditional medicine. They would express their frustrations about how the medical system had failed them when they needed help the most. Mary took the time to listen to their problems. Some patients came because even though their medications helped their primary syndrome, the side effects became too much to bear. Mary listened to them all with an open mind and compassionate understanding of their frustrations. Often, it seemed as though she could anticipate what her patients needed.

Mary was clearly the most successful practitioner in her group. Yet it wasn't because she had the most experience or the highest grades in her nursing classes. It was because she would pull up a chair and listen to her patients' stories. She paid close attention and treated patients in a compassionate, nonjudgmental way. For the first time in their journey through the medical system, they felt heard. Mary's compassionate presence helped many people on their way to good health.

Compassion is the willingness to acknowledge and be moved by the suffering of others. The word "compassion" has roots in the Latin words *pati* and *cum*, which mean "to suffer with." Compassion includes a desire to help those who are suffering, as well as an attitude of nonjudgment. When you offer true compassion to your patients, they feel listened to, cared for, appreciated, and understood.

The medical profession has always recognized the importance of compassion—governmental programs teach it, researchers study it, and hospitals give patients questionnaires asking how well their nurses practiced it. Without compassion, how could you spend your days caring for scarred bodies, exhausted minds, and people struggling with a fear of death?

Consider This:

Do you consider yourself to be a compassionate nurse? Do you wish there was more you could do for a patient than just give them prescribed medications? Have you ever left a patient's room feeling guilty because they wanted to talk and you had to excuse yourself because you had other work that needed to be done? Have you ever held the hand of a dying patient and felt peace, not sadness, after their passing?

Compassion pushes you—as a healthcare provider—out of bed in the morning with enough oomph to manage your day. By practicing compassion, you are changing the world. After all, compassion, as the Dalai Lama says, radiates to others…and science agrees!

In a staged experiment conducted at Northeastern University, psychologists discovered that people who felt compassion for one person treated others with more compassion.[26] To put it another way, if you feel compassion for the long-suffering cancer survivor, you're likely to feel less resentment toward the hypochondriac down the hall.

Nurses are compassionate people. Indeed, the compassion you feel for others may be one of the main reasons you chose nursing as your profession. Doctors might whiz by on rounds, but nurses are always there to care for those who are suffering. Ninety percent of participants in a 2011 World Health Organization study cited the desire to care for and help people as their main reason for choosing a career in nursing.[27]

Impact of Compassion

Communication is an important aspect of any interaction. Compassionate communication is especially important in the healthcare profession where people are surrounded by suffering. And it's particularly important when you need to be the bearer of bad news.

Compassion is often defined as an action undertaken with sensitivity to the needs of others, a purposeful and voluntary action to foster the well-being of others. It is a key part of the Hippocratic Oath: "I will remember that…warmth, sympathy, and understanding may outweigh the surgeon's knife or the chemist's drug." Compassion is clearly a tremendously important ingredient in taking care of people, and science has demonstrated the power of compassion to heal. For example, the Dignity Health and Center for Compassion and Altruism Research and Education (CCARE) found that treating patients with compassion led to positive health effects. These effects included reduced pain, lowered anxiety and blood pressure, faster wound healing, and shorter hospital stays.[28] Studies have also shown that patients are more than twice as likely to follow the advice of a doctor who is a good, compassionate communicator. What's more, surgical patients healed faster and left the hospital sooner when anesthesiologists encouraged them post-op. Also, when patients were approached with compassion, they felt more engaged in their own care and were more motivated to give important information to their doctors that could lead to more accurate diagnoses and better treatment.[29]

Compassion is born within the depths of our being.
It arises as a deep stirring beneath the mud of our everyday mind.
What stirs it is the force of motivation and commitment
to engage with our pain and the pain of others.
—*Mindful Compassion,* by Paul Gilbert and Choden

The positive effects of compassion are not restricted to patients. Rather, the benefits flow both ways. Research has shown that compassionate care benefits medical staff because it creates a working atmosphere where employees feel less exhausted and more engaged. This is no small matter for nurses who struggle with long work hours and high stress levels.[30]

For anyone ready to dismiss compassion and its effects as "pseudoscientific" or elusive, science indicates otherwise. Researchers have begun to map the biological basis of compassion. Studies show that when people are compassionate, their heart rates slow down and oxytocin—the bonding hormone—is released. Feeling compassion activates the brain areas associated with pleasurable feelings. Simply put, showing compassion to others makes us feel good!

Have you ever wondered why you feel like crying when you see someone else in tears? Or why you recoil reflexively when you see someone on the street get hit by a random object? Early research shows that brain cells called "mirror" neurons provide the neurological basis for the ability to identify and feel what others are feeling.[31] The implications are far-reaching. It has been proposed, for example, that mirror neurons play an important role in social development, in learning, and in practicing compassion.

Nurse Olivia Traynor's experience is a good illustration of the importance of compassion in nursing. Olivia was the director of nursing for a busy rehabilitation hospital. She took pride in ensuring her workers were happy and her patients received the highest level of care. Her nursing facility often needed to recruit more nurses. Angie, a recent graduate, came to Olivia looking for a job. The interview went well, and Olivia was excited to have such a talented nurse on her unit.

As Angie settled into her new role, Olivia got a sense that all was not well. After Angie joined the team, colleagues would say things were fine but would look away when Olivia asked how things were going. Olivia suspected they were not telling the entire truth. Finally, she decided to discuss the new hire with the charge nurse. The charge nurse told Olivia that Angie seemed to have trouble accepting her role. In particular, she often snapped at patients and seemed anxious about everything. Often, she seemed eager to get her work over and done with quickly and leave the building at the earliest opportunity. On top of that, she tended to avoid certain tasks, which made her coworkers less than enthusiastic to work with her.

Olivia knew she had to step in, but she wasn't sure how. Berating Angie or telling her to change her ways wouldn't solve the problem. Certainly, that would only make this new nurse feel worse. No, she realized, something was wrong here, something beyond mere discipline. When Olivia eventually called Angie into the office, the look in the new grad's eyes was one of abject terror. However, instead of reprimanding, Olivia smiled at her. When asked how she liked her new role, Angie could not control her tears.

As she sobbed, Angie disclosed how much stress she felt trying to adapt to her new career. She felt it was all too much for her, that she had made a terrible mistake in choosing nursing. When Angie stopped talking, Olivia let silence hang in the air. After a few moments, Olivia told Angie that she, too, had struggled in her first nursing job, and that it had been difficult to find her way and keep up with the heavy workload. As Olivia spoke, all the tension Angie had been holding for weeks dissolved. She felt a deep sense of relief, realizing that Olivia understood.

Through Olivia's compassionate approach to this troubled new nurse, they were able to find a way that the new grad could work through her difficulties and become the nurse that she always wanted to be. Together, the two nurses explored their goals and ways Olivia could help Angie work toward them. As the weeks went by, Olivia saw Angie blossom on the unit, and her coworkers had high praise for her. Instead of reprimanding her, the director had treated her with compassion. Subsequently, the two talked weekly about how Angie was holding up in the face of so many challenges. In time, Angie became an excellent nurse and learned to extend to her patients the same compassion she had received.

Mindfulness and Compassion

Angie had a difficult start but learned a valuable lesson about the reciprocity of compassion—the more she received, the more she was able to give. She also learned the value of having compassion not just for others, but also for herself. Research over the last two decades has consistently shown that mindfulness increases empathy and compassion for ourselves and others.[32]

The Building Blocks of Compassion

Compassion is not simply an emotion, and it depends on much more than traits such as kindness and warmth. Rather, as the work of psychologist Paul Gilbert and his colleague Choden has shown, compassion is dependent on a complex combination of certain skills and abilities.[33]

As you read through the following qualities that underpin compassion, see if you can relate to them in terms of how you engage emotionally when you encounter distress in others.

The Six Compassion Attributes

1. *Motivation.* Without motivation, you cannot engage with or alleviate suffering. Motivation stems from a desire to be caring and helpful to others; you are invested in their well-being and want to do something to alleviate their distress. Olivia needed motivation to alleviate Angie's distress.

2. *Sensitivity.* Sensitivity helps you notice that the other person is distressed. If you lack sensitivity, you may turn a blind eye when others need your help, rationalizing and justifying your behavior. If Olivia were not able to be sensitive to and in tune with Angie's feelings, she would not have been able to help her.

3. *Sympathy.* Sensitivity inclines you toward having sympathy for others. When you have sympathy, you feel moved by the distress in yourself and others and motivated to alleviate it. Without this urge to help, compassion is not possible. Olivia's sympathy for Angie compelled her to reach out.

4. *Nonjudgment.* Acceptance allows you to accept the person in their distress, rather than blame or judge them. Nonjudgment is a mindfulness skill. It allowed Olivia to reflect wisely on Angie's dilemma and not blame her.

5. *Empathy.* When you feel empathy, you can make sense of the other person's feelings and your own emotional response. Rather than becoming angry with Angie for not doing her job properly, Olivia was able to empathize with her struggles and help her. Empathy is the bridge between engaging with and alleviating suffering. For example, if you were treating a patient whose carelessness had harmed himself and others, it would be easy to become angry at his thoughtlessness. However, empathizing with his shame and guilt would help you be more compassionate and effective in his treatment.

6. *Distress Tolerance.* When you have distress tolerance, you are able to bear your own difficult feelings and those of others. By contrast, sympathy might trigger a distressing emotional response. For example, Olivia could have just as easily become so distressed and overwhelmed by Angie's struggles at work that she would have been unable to help her. Fortunately for Angie, Olivia was able to tolerate her own feelings and be with Angie in her distress. Because she wasn't sidetracked by her own or Angie's distress, Olivia was able to engage and take productive steps to offer relief.

Journal Reflection:

Bring to mind a time when you were moved by the distress of another person and wanted to help them. From the rich tapestry of compassion attributes discussed above, name any qualities you felt in that situation. Were any attributes missing? How did the presence or absence of these qualities affect your response to the person who was distressed?

You may be able to access the compassionate qualities of motivation, sensitivity, sympathy, nonjudgment, empathy, and distress tolerance quite naturally in your everyday interactions. However, when you are stressed, tired, or overworked, this might change. If you are constantly bombarded with too many conflicting demands in a stressed, understaffed healthcare facility, it may be harder for you to access empathy, tolerate the distress you see around you, and slow down sufficiently to engage compassionately. That is why it is important to train in compassion. Doing so will build your capacity to engage heartfully when you are weary, and work in a high-demand environment that is challenging, unpredictable, and stressed.

Emergence of Compassion

The real compassion test is how we behave when we are stressed, rushed, hassled, and no one is watching.

—Aidan Halligan

Taken together, the six compassion attributes help us tune into suffering, understand it, and tolerate it. Each attribute interconnects with and influences the other. For example, when you practice sensitivity, you enhance sympathy. In turn, when you practice sympathy, you enhance empathy. When you practice empathy, you improve distress tolerance. Like interlocking, supporting bricks in a structure, your edifice will be stronger when all the bricks are in place.

Imagine you are a nurse working in the ER when a male victim of a nasty car accident is rushed into the unit accompanied by his wife. She is physically unharmed but emotional and distraught. Clearly, she has the motivation to engage with his suffering, in that she is incredibly sympathetic and instinctively can imagine how he is feeling. However, she is overwhelmed, frightened, consumed with anger, and blames the other driver in the accident. All she can feel is her spouse's pain and her own anger and anxiety. She has no distress tolerance. In other words, although she can feel her husband's pain, she can do nothing to alleviate it. Similarly, she can also feel her own suffering, but it overwhelms her; she is unable to do anything to alleviate her distress or offer comfort to her husband.

By contrast, as a trained, mindful nurse, you are motivated to respond to your patient's suffering. Because of this, you are sensitive to it, and while you experience an initial sympathy response, you don't become overwhelmed. Rather than judging or blaming, you remain focused, manage your emotions, empathize, and understand. As a result, you can manage your distress and focus on the next phase of compassion, which is to alleviate the suffering.

Journal Reflection:

If you were to focus on strengthening one of these qualities, which one would you choose? For example, do you need to develop your empathy or become more able to bear your own emotions or those of others?

Compassionate Skills

These six emotional qualities are essential for you to engage your compassion. Nevertheless, if you feel lacking in any of these attributes, don't worry: each quality can be cultivated in the course of your everyday life. Every nursing interaction offers an opportunity to practice the six attributes.

Compassion and mindfulness interact, and the practice of mindfulness enhances compassionate qualities. Mindfulness facilitates compassion, like the catalyst of a chemical reaction. By developing a sense of interconnectedness and establishing emotional control, mindfulness nourishes development of the six compassion attributes and protects you from being paralyzed by another person's distress. By cultivating nonjudgment, mindfulness helps you to understand the causes of suffering. And by sharpening focus, mindfulness allows you to attend to what is necessary to take compassionate action.

GRACE

To practice compassion in clinical encounters, Roshi Joan Halifax developed what she called the GRACE practice, designed for people who work in stressful environments.[34] A simple mnemonic that is easy to remember, GRACE offers an easy-to-use practice to open up to your patients' experiences while staying centered in the here and now. It helps you to develop the capacity for an effective compassionate response.

As you interact with your patient, this practice helps you to slow down and become more aware—and creates fertile soil so that compassion can arise. It contains five elements, each involving important processes:

Try This:
GRACE Practice

G—Gather your attention. Take time at the beginning of the interaction to focus, breathe, and be present. Use this time to minimize distractions and mental clutter, and allow yourself to be present in the here and now. Narrow your focus to a single sensation, such as your breathing, or focus on the soles of your feet or on your hands to re-center yourself. Gathering your attention in this way allows you to be fully present.

R—Recall your intention. Take a moment to reconnect with your core values and motivations, as well as your desire to truly help the person with whom you are in contact. It's too easy in a busy, hectic workplace to lose connection with the higher purpose of your actions. For instance, when you give meds or reassure a patient, you may see these encounters as routine elements of your workday. If you do that, however, your job becomes mundane and disconnected from its true meaning.

(cont'd)

A—Attune to yourself and the other person. Once you gain emotional control and focus, turn your attention to the person you are with. Attend to your patient with the intention to fully understand them, and hear what they are saying. Observe their body language and nonverbal signs such as their tone of voice. Being fully attentive enhances your sensitivity and maximizes your compassionate action.

C—Consider what is truly helpful for the person. Avoid automatically going with the first action that comes into your mind and, instead, challenge yourself to be open and attend to how the patient is presenting. What are you sensing? Where is that coming from? What does it really mean? Use your knowledge and experience, rather than assumptions and habits, to determine possible actions.

E—Engage and enact. Effective compassionate action is now possible; in the form of a recommendation you make or an action you take. Because of the mutual trust developed from your genuine desire to help, the 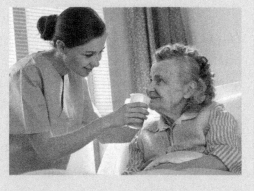 patient is more likely to accept your recommendation.

The "E" in GRACE also stands for *Ending* the interaction in a focused, positive way. Recognize when the encounter is complete, so you can frame it appropriately for both the patient and yourself. That way, you set accurate expectations and free yourself to move to your next encounter, without the burden of unfinished business. This closure allows you to repeat the GRACE practice with your next patient.

Journal Reflection:

Imagine a scenario where you are interacting with a patient. In what ways might GRACE improve this interaction? Reflect on the compassionate attributes you use in the GRACE practice.

Developing Compassion

Given the nature of your work—you're dealing daily with suffering—it is important that you understand what compassion is and how to strengthen it. Hopefully, this chapter has given you a sense of the multifaceted qualities you can draw on to nurture your compassionate instinct. It may seem like a lot to remember, but try not to feel overwhelmed with the details! Subsequent chapters will help you develop these attributes through various practices, and in time they will become intuitive and part of your way of being.

Compassion arises from inside you—it is already present within you like a seed that needs to be cultivated. If you feed and water it, your compassion will grow—and so will you. Yet, a person cannot achieve becoming and staying compassionate overnight. It is a process, a skill, and like mindfulness, it takes time and practice. The rewards can be life-changing.

Practice Plan:

Take some time to digest the material explored in this chapter and to reflect on your experience of compassion in your nursing practice. Begin using the GRACE practice in your everyday interactions to help strengthen your compassionate presence. Notice if your interactions change in any way. Continue to practice mindful movement, alternating it with sitting meditation and mindful walking.

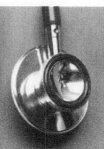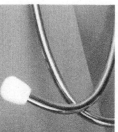

Points to Remember

+ Compassion is a feeling of concern for the suffering of others and the wish to alleviate it.
+ Studies indicate that the practice of compassion benefits both staff and patients.
+ Research shows that mindfulness helps improve your compassion capacity by helping you feel interconnected, empathetic, and more focused on others.
+ Compassion comprises several attributes which support each other, and when they function properly, these form the core of compassion.
+ The GRACE practice helps you to express compassion during patient encounters.

CHAPTER TWELVE

The Constant Giver: Compassion Fatigue

The expectation that we can be immersed in suffering and loss daily and not be touched by it is as unrealistic as expecting to be able to walk through water without getting wet.
—Rachel Naomi Remen

Sally worked as a staff nurse on the oncology ward of a busy hospital. She found her shifts increasingly difficult and often felt tearful and anxious. In particular, she felt frustrated and angry about not being able to offer more help to patients and families. Sometimes Sally talked of leaving the ward and moving to a less emotionally charged working environment. When she felt overwhelmed by sadness and negativity, she called in sick and spent a day in bed, too exhausted to go out or meet a friend.

Sally was experiencing compassion fatigue. Although she was unaware of it, this affected her personal and professional life. She was unfamiliar with strategies to combat compassion fatigue, yet with the right actions and support, she could have achieved a healthy balance and found a way to be content in her job.

Consider This:

Have you called in sick on more than one occasion because you felt unable to cope with another day at work? When is the last time you enjoyed a good laugh, or smiled so hard your face hurt? Do you suffer sudden chest pains or heart palpitations while at work? When is the last time you had a restful night's sleep? Do you withdraw from patients experiencing severe pain, where once you would have sat by their side for as long as you were needed?

Defining Compassion Fatigue

Joinson was the first to describe *compassion fatigue* as a form of burnout that affects people in the caring professions.[35] Particularly common in nurses who deal daily with pain and death, compassion fatigue has been described as "a heavy heart, accompanied with debilitating weariness, brought on by the everyday empathetic responses to the pain and suffering experienced by others in the nurse's care."[36]

At work you offer yourself as a therapeutic tool. Interactions with patients and compassionate behaviors can help make your patients feel better, but this can be extremely taxing for you, especially if you don't take enough care to replenish the energy you constantly, generously give others.

Anywhere from 40% to 85% of helping professionals suffer from compassion fatigue or exhibit trauma symptoms. Some specialties—including palliative care, oncology, pediatrics, and traumatology—are more prone to this problem.[37]

Many things, ranging from moody and unenthusiastic coworkers to the overwhelming demands of the overstretched healthcare system, can sap your energy. Amid all the chaos and rush is the patient. Most of all, you want to be there for the patient who presents with pain, distress, fear, and a mix of heavyweight emotions.

People who gravitate toward nursing typically do so because they have personality traits that favor caring for and nurturing others. But when a nurse constantly puts the needs and feelings of others first, she may neglect her own needs—especially if she doesn't take time to build herself up again after an exhausting stint at work.

Compassion fatigue is easily missed, or masked as something else. Nurse Sally tried to brush her discomfort aside, attributing her emotions to a bad day at work. Yet her recurring headaches, sadness, and frequent sickness were signs of compassion fatigue. What at first appears to be a harmless and temporary hiccup in a nurse's mental and physical health can develop into a chronic condition. In extreme cases, compassion fatigue can lead to self-destructive behaviors, addictions, and even suicide.

The Diagnostic and Statistical Manual of Mental Disorders now lists compassion fatigue as a type of post-traumatic stress disorder, which means that working with people in trauma can affect you as deeply as spending time in a war zone.[38]

Burned Out or Loved Out?

Does compassion fatigue equal burnout? Not quite, although there is overlap between them, and some symptoms are common to both. Burnout in nursing can occur after years spent absorbing the physical and emotional trauma of many patients, combined with a sense of one's own helplessness. The result of long-term work-related issues and on-going stress, burnout usually has a slow and pernicious onset.

By contrast, compassion fatigue often strikes suddenly and delivers a knockout punch. It can result from one particular event or long-term exposure to the suffering of others. A nurse who is burned out is more likely to develop compassion fatigue. In *Countering Compassion Fatigue: A Requisite Nursing Agenda*, Deborah Boyle noted another difference between the two phenomena: "While the burnt-out nurse gradually withdraws, the compassionately fatigued nurse tries harder to give even more to patients in need. Both outcomes, however, are associated with a sense of depletion within the nurse, a running-on-empty feeling."[39]

Test Yourself

The following is a list of symptoms most commonly associated with compassion fatigue.[40] You may want to check off those that apply to you as the starting point in figuring out whether you might need a psychological nip and tuck.

Work-Related

- ☐ Avoidance or dread of working with certain patients
- ☐ Reduced ability to feel empathy toward patients or families
- ☐ Frequent use of sick days
- ☐ Lack of joyfulness

Physical

- ☐ Headaches
- ☐ Digestive problems (such as diarrhea, constipation, upset stomach)
- ☐ Muscle tension
- ☐ Sleep disturbances (such as inability to sleep, insomnia, too much sleep)
- ☐ Fatigue
- ☐ Cardiac symptoms (such as chest pain/pressure, palpitations, tachycardia)

Emotional

- ☐ Mood swings
- ☐ Restlessness
- ☐ Irritability
- ☐ Oversensitivity
- ☐ Anxiety
- ☐ Excessive use of substances (such as nicotine, alcohol, illicit or prescribed drugs)
- ☐ Depression
- ☐ Anger and resentment
- ☐ Loss of objectivity
- ☐ Memory issues
- ☐ Poor concentration, focus, and judgment

Any one of these symptoms could indicate you suffer from compassion fatigue, but people with this condition generally exhibit more than one symptom.

Do you think you might be suffering from compassion fatigue? If so, you can assess your level using the Professional Quality of Life self-test in Appendix B.[41]

Nurses tend to absorb and internalize the emotions of clients and, at times, coworkers, making the pain of others their own.

—Christina Melvin

Empathetic Distress or Compassion Fatigue?

The care you provide as a nurse is often based on an empathetic relationship between you and your patients. Empathy, however, doesn't equal compassion. To prevent compassion fatigue, it is important to distinguish between the two.

Although empathy is a precursor to feeling compassion, it is not necessarily a positive thing. Brain scans have shown that when you feel empathy for someone, the same areas of your brain are activated as in the brain of the sufferer. As a result, empathy hurts; you internalize the person's pain and feel it as though you were going through it yourself. Over time, unmanaged empathy stimulates negative emotions, such as acute sadness, anger, and fear, and it can easily lead to distress.

What's more, empathy can be antisocial, triggering an urge to isolate and avoid contact with others. When this happens, nurses are no longer able to make a genuine connection with their patients. Instead, they are overwhelmed by trying to avoid their own collapse under the strain of difficult emotions.

Compassion, on the other hand, is a warm and loving emotion that does not involve feeling what the other person is feeling. Although you acknowledge their sadness and pain, it doesn't become *your* pain.

When you feel compassion, your brain fires along different pathways, and rather than feeling the distress of others, positive caring emotions are engendered. Compassion is about the *action* and brings a strong motivation to help or make a difference. When you transform empathy into compassion, you don't become overwhelmed.

In the next two chapters, you will learn loving-kindness and other compassion practices that protect you from distress by activating warm, nurturing feelings inside you when you're faced with suffering in yourself or others.

> *Without the support of love and compassion, empathy by itself is like an electric pump through which no water circulates, and it will quickly overheat and burn. Empathy should take place within the much vaster space of altruistic love.*

—Matthieu Ricard

Because true compassion does not lead to fatigue, many argue that the widely used term "compassion fatigue" is a misnomer, and should be changed to "empathetic fatigue". When you start sinking, what you experience is empathetic fatigue. What's more, it can be remedied by cultivating love and compassion. Compassion builds strength, resilience, and the capacity to relieve suffering. And unlike empathy, it does not become worn.

Switching from empathy to compassion has profound benefits for you, your nursing practice, and your patients. In particular, compassion helps you move from a potentially negative mode to a deeply positive and empowering one. When you take a compassionate stance when confronted with suffering, you can offer help effectively while also preserving your own inner balance and strength, and remain healthy and well. Instead of dwelling on the negativity of it all, you can develop healthy boundaries to ensure that pain and grief do not overpower you.

Often we feel that silence and stillness aren't good enough when suffering is present. We feel compelled to 'do something': to talk, console, work, clean, move around, 'help.' But in the shared embrace of meditation, a caregiver and dying person can be held in an intimate silence beyond consolation or assistance.

—Joan Halifax

A compassionate nurse is able to be present, to listen, and to care. Even when you feel there is nothing more you can do for a patient, you can still provide compassion, connect with the person, and know you have made a difference. Instead of shutting down in the face of suffering that you cannot cure, you can choose to stay present. Christie Lane, in the following excerpt from her journal article, writes movingly about mindful presence as a compassionate act. Like her, you can find the nurturing love and resilience inside you and engage.

"One evening I cared for a woman whose cancer had spread throughout her body. Although she had already been given her ordered dose of pain medication, she woke during the night with terrible spasms of pain racking her body. She told me that she had never experienced the pain as being so severe. Having already given her the maximum dose of pain medication ordered, I paged the doctor on call. At that moment, I felt somewhat useless, and then I remembered the significance of being present, so I simply stood

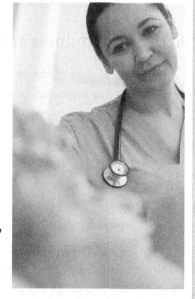

there at her bedside holding her hand as she wailed in pain. I did not speak; I did not move except to occasionally touch her head. I did not run from her room to escape the misery of her moans; I remained silent and still. The violent spasms of pain subsided shortly after additional doses of medication were given; but it was my presence that she repeatedly thanked me for, not the drugs. She told me how grateful she was that I had stayed calmly by her side. It can be very trying to witness the suffering of another, but that presence has power. In that moment, in the stillness of presence, there is a coming together; there is true love and compassion."[42]

Journal Reflection:

Bring to mind a situation in your nursing career when you shared your healing, compassionate presence with a patient. How did you feel being fully present? How do you feel now, recalling this experience?

Practice Mindfulness and Compassion

The state of compassion is whole and sustaining;
the compassionate mind is not broken or shattered by
facing states of suffering. It is spacious and resilient.
—Sharon Salzberg

Mindfulness and compassion are antidotes to compassion fatigue. Engaging in these practices alters brain activity, gradually reducing activity in the brain areas associated with negative feelings, thus preventing onset of this condition. You can change the physiology and structure of your brain by cultivating compassion and become better equipped for the everyday challenges of your work. As a result, symptoms of stress and mood disturbances will be replaced with healthy reactions that nurture your well-being and increase your capacity for compassionate care.

Recognize Compassion Fatigue

Compassion fatigue is an under-recognized phenomenon, and awareness is the key to recovery.

A nurse who develops compassion fatigue is often unable to see or sense the gradually increasing problem. There may be subtle signs at first, such as not taking the time to listen to a patient's concerns or rushing through a painful procedure. Someone else—a colleague or nurse manager—may be the first to spot the telltale signs.

Earlier in this chapter, you read about Sally, who worked on a busy oncology ward. Sally did not want her manager to know she was struggling. Especially, she didn't want to be labeled as someone who couldn't cut it or wasn't capable of being a professional nurse. Yet she found it hard just to get out of bed in the morning, and when she finally managed to drag herself to work, she felt anxious and unable to focus. Still, she persevered, showing up day after day, going through the motions, feeling irritable and tired, and just getting through the routine. Her manager had a limited awareness of compassion fatigue as an occupational hazard. Unfortunately, her facility had not invested time or funding resources to raise compassion fatigue awareness among nurses and managers. Finally, Sally transferred to labor and delivery, hoping that participating in the happy event of new life would help her feel better.

For a few weeks after her transfer, Sally felt more energized. She put her earlier problem down to the strain of her work in oncology, experiencing the grief of so many terminally ill patients and not being able to change things for the better. However, the feelings of hopelessness and anxiety crept back, leaving her just as miserable as she had been before. Once again, she dreaded going to work. She was tired all the time, started drinking to compensate for her feelings, and ended up divorcing her husband because she felt he wasn't providing the support she needed.

Even before Sally transferred from oncology to labor and delivery, she was suffering from compassion fatigue. Without proper intervention and support, it was only a matter of time before her difficult feelings would resurface and the spiral would begin all over again.

One of Sally's friends was a nurse in a different facility, and they often talked together about how Sally felt. In time, her friend revealed that she had suffered compassion fatigue in the past and recommended Sally research it. When Sally saw the symptom list, she checked all the boxes. For the first time, she had a label that helped her understand her plight. She knew, however, that the help she needed was not available through her facility, so she researched privately for a therapist who specialized in compassion fatigue. Through her sessions with the therapist, Sally learned how to implement self-care, set boundaries, and restore balance in her life. Whenever she saw nurses on her unit struggling with the same problem, she would educate them about compassion fatigue. Although Sally didn't get the support she needed from her facility to help her through her own journey, she was able to help other struggling nurses.

Mindfulness helps you to identify and deal with the early warning signs of compassion fatigue before it has a chance to escalate. Unfortunately, Sally's case was full blown before she sought professional help. With the help of mindfulness, you can tune in to subtle changes in your mood and behavior, and ask for support before things get out of hand.

A research study[43] investigating compassion fatigue in nurses revealed that it was often triggered by patient care situations in which nurses:

- Believed that their actions would "not make a difference" or "never seemed to be enough".

- Experienced problems with the system (high patient census, heavy patient assignments, high acuity, overtime, and extra workdays).
- Had personal issues, such as inexperience or inadequate energy.
- Identified with the patients.
- Overlooked serious patient symptoms.

Preventing Compassion Fatigue

Compassion fatigue is a common phenomenon, and nurses are especially vulnerable. This is alarming, considering its serious impact on nurses' well-being and patient care. The important take-home message is this: You can take steps to avoid driving yourself to the point of exhaustion. In particular, you need to become aware of your behaviors and the physical and emotional states that make you vulnerable to compassion fatigue and burnout. When you feel fatigue and distress creeping up and threatening to move into red-zone levels, you need to ramp up your self-care.

With the help of the compassion practices you will learn in the next two chapters, the symptoms of burnout and fatigue will lessen. Your ability to cope with your workdays will recharge, firing up healthy compassion toward patients and families. This can free you to focus on your patients' immediate crises and help you to respond calmly, while minimizing risks to your health and well-being.

Practice Plan:

This week, notice your personal boundaries at work. If you find yourself overextending and feeling what your patients are possibly feeling (fear, sadness, or grief), practice shifting your attention away from the difficult emotions and back to your body and breath. Re-engage after you have centered yourself.

To help you stay grounded, continue to alternate or mix the formal practices of mindful movement, walking meditations, and sitting meditations. Follow fifteen minutes of walking meditation with fifteen minutes of mindful movement one day, and the next day try fifteen minutes of sitting meditation followed by fifteen minutes of movement.

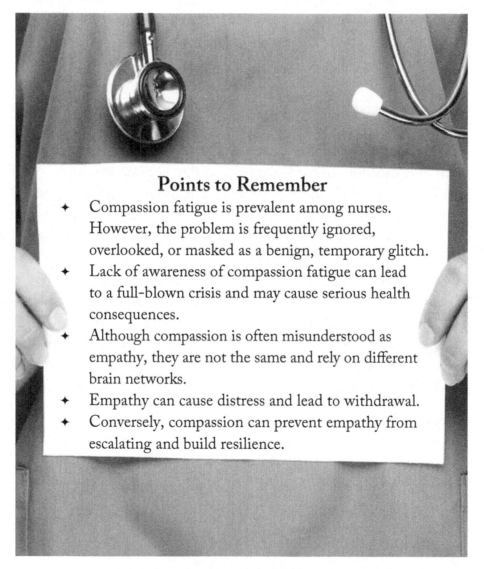

Points to Remember

+ Compassion fatigue is prevalent among nurses. However, the problem is frequently ignored, overlooked, or masked as a benign, temporary glitch.
+ Lack of awareness of compassion fatigue can lead to a full-blown crisis and may cause serious health consequences.
+ Although compassion is often misunderstood as empathy, they are not the same and rely on different brain networks.
+ Empathy can cause distress and lead to withdrawal.
+ Conversely, compassion can prevent empathy from escalating and build resilience.

CHAPTER THIRTEEN

Cultivating Self-Compassion

Compassion for others begins with kindness to ourselves.
—Pema Chödrön

Mindfulness can untangle you from the most pathological side effects of compassion fatigue. When you regain your balance and decide to reconnect, you need to focus your attention on self-compassion.

Self-compassion is the capacity for healthy nurturing of the self. Just as compassion is the willingness to acknowledge and be moved by the suffering of others, self-compassion extends this acceptance and care to *you*. As the antidote to compassion fatigue, self-compassion is essential for nurses. After all, just like on an airplane, if you don't put on your "oxygen mask" first, then you won't be able to help anyone else. The development of self-compassion is necessary if you are to provide sustained compassionate care for others.

A nurse named Debbie struggled with self-compassion. Debbie was a part-time IV-team nurse who also worked telemetry. Her IV-team job required her to help floor nurses start IVs for patients with challenging veins. Most of her patients were in pain and not always grateful to the nurses who helped them. Debbie felt for them. She understood the pain these patients felt and attempted to help them any way she could, such as wrapping their arms in hot towels, using smaller-gauge needles, and only using the tourniquet as long as necessary. She would also sit at their bedsides and listen to how they were feeling long after she had successfully inserted the IV. Some patients were scared, some in pain, others ready for the new challenges ahead. One open-heart surgery patient could not stop crying because, over the course of many hospitalizations, her arms had developed scar tissue from so many IVs. No matter how busy Debbie was, she took time to listen as her patients shared their fears and concerns. Her compassion levels exceeded that of many of her colleagues.

One night, exhausted and overwhelmed after working an intense twelve-hour shift on telemetry, Debbie missed the lab results for a patient with a known history of high potassium due to kidney failure. A routine blood test was run in the morning.

A lab technician called her with the elevated result, but, in Debbie's opinion, it wasn't high enough to warrant immediate action, such as calling for the rapid-response team. Still, she wanted to call the doctor to get orders for a medication that would lower the potassium, but before she could make the call, one of her other patients had a fall. Debbie got so caught up in this emergency that she completely forgot about the patient with the elevated potassium. Meantime, the potassium level continued to rise, and, as the shift was ending, the patient coded.

Debbie was devastated about her oversight. She failed to act in time, even though she knew this patient was at risk. No matter how hard she tried, she couldn't stop thinking about it. How could she be so stupid? How could she let herself be distracted from something so important? Although Debbie was written up for failing to act, her manager was understanding and discussed ways to prevent similar life-threatening situations in the future. Even though her manager reassured Debbie that mistakes happen and the patient was fine now, Debbie continued to beat herself up. No matter how hard she tried, she couldn't get it out of her mind. In her eyes, she had failed terribly as a nurse. For days, she criticized herself so much that she could barely focus on her work. If Debbie's colleague had made the same mistake, Debbie would have been the first to offer comfort and reassurance, but she could not comfort herself because she didn't think she deserved it after such an obvious error. The compassion she so generously gave to others was in short supply when it came to herself.

How much self-compassion do you possess? Picture yourself tripping up at work as Debbie did. Let's say you arrived late, failed to get everything done, or said the wrong thing. Do you attack yourself for every little imperfection? You might say to yourself, "How could I have been so stupid?" or "Why can't I ever accomplish as much in a shift as the other nurses?"

These judgments cycle through your mind and stir up stress. In an attempt to halt the pain, you berate yourself, and your stress escalates. Although the thoughts and feelings are uncomfortable, you continue to condemn yourself long after the event, creating even more stress for yourself.

Remember the three components of stress we examined in Chapter 9? We talked about how stress is a cycle of physical tension, painful emotions, and rumination. All three were triggered for Debbie following her error. Fortunately, self-compassion offers the key to breaking that cycle.

Avoiding Self-Attacks

When you fling insults at yourself, your inner critic takes over. This quickly ramps up your anxiety levels and activates the fight-or-flight response. Distracted and self-critical, you think about what happened, tossing it around in your mind, and going over it again and again. Lost in reactivity, you lose sight of the need to treat yourself kindly.

Because you are both the attacker and the attacked, your body floods with the stress hormone cortisol. Over time, this flood causes mental and physical damage and impairs your health, your sleep, your ability to think clearly, and your ability to function competently at work.

Consider This:

Do you feel guilty for taking a sick day, whether it is for physical or emotional needs? Do you constantly criticize yourself for not being able to give patients one-on-one care, as often as they need or desire it? Do you continue to blame yourself even after you have been forgiven by others? Do you constantly berate yourself for not being perfect, or for not having all the right answers all of the time?

The remedy when things go wrong is to step outside that pull of self-judgment and practice self-compassion instead. Rather than berating yourself when you slip up, be gentle. Speak kindly to yourself and accept what has happened. This doesn't mean that you let yourself off the hook for your error. Indeed, it's the opposite. When you are self-compassionate, you are more likely to own up to what happened. Turning toward your distress with compassion helps you to let go of defensiveness. Rather than judging yourself, you can now acknowledge difficult feelings such as guilt and shame. This frees up energy so that you can look for helpful solutions to your dilemma and focus on how to avoid repeating what went wrong.

If your compassion doesn't include yourself, it is incomplete.

—Jack Kornfield

Self-Compassion Soothes Painful Emotions

Self-compassion helps you recognize and soothe your painful thoughts and emotions. When you identify and relate to your emotions with kindness instead of harshness, you tap into your biological caregiving system. Oxytocin, the feel-good hormone, is released, which helps you feel calm, comforted, and secure.

With practice, you can relate to your fears and anxieties with compassionate understanding, just as you might relate to a patient. Self-compassion is yours to tap into at any moment when you acknowledge that your nature is inherently good and that you deserve a generous dose of self-value and self-gratitude. When you carry these mindfulness treatments in your metaphorical IV-bag, you can inject yourself with a fresh dose of confidence and competence to fight off depression and anxiety. This will help you to move through challenging circumstances during your shift with greater and greater ease.

Nurses truly embrace the value of compassionate care when they treat themselves compassionately.

—— *Taking Time for Support,* by Marlene Z. Cohen,
Katherine Brown-Saltzman, and Marilyn J. Shirk

How Self-Compassionate Are You?

How do you rate yourself in terms of self-compassion? Dr. Kirsten Neff, a psychologist at the University of Texas, devised a scale to measure how much self-compassion a person has.[44] The shortened version of Neff's scale that appears below was reformatted by the Psychology Department, Ohio State University.

Read each statement carefully before answering and check off how often you behave in the way described. (See the points for each answer immediately below each checkbox and note how the scoring is not the same for each answer. Items followed by the letter 'R' indicate reverse scores).

Please respond to each item by marking one box per row		Never	Rarely	Sometimes	Often	Always
1	When I fail at something important to me I become consumed by feelings of inadequacy. (R)	☐ 5	☐ 4	☐ 3	☐ 2	☐ 1
2	I try to be understanding and patient towards those aspects of my personality I don't like.	☐ 1	☐ 2	☐ 3	☐ 4	☐ 5
3	When something painful happens I try to take a balanced view of the situation.	☐ 1	☐ 2	☐ 3	☐ 4	☐ 5
4	When I'm feeling down, I tend to feel like most other people are probably happier than I am. (R)	☐ 5	☐ 4	☐ 3	☐ 2	☐ 1
5	I try to see my failings as part of the human condition.	☐ 1	☐ 2	☐ 3	☐ 4	☐ 5
6	When I'm going through a very hard time, I give myself the caring and tenderness I need.	☐ 1	☐ 2	☐ 3	☐ 4	☐ 5
7	When something upsets me I try to keep my emotions in balance.	☐ 1	☐ 2	☐ 3	☐ 4	☐ 5
8	When I fail at something that's important to me I tend to feel alone in my failure. (R)	☐ 5	☐ 4	☐ 3	☐ 2	☐ 1
9	When I'm feeling down I tend to obsess and fixate on everything that's wrong. (R)	☐ 5	☐ 4	☐ 3	☐ 2	☐ 1
10	When I feel inadequate in some way, I try to remind myself that feelings of inadequacy are shared by most people.	☐ 1	☐ 2	☐ 3	☐ 4	☐ 5
11	I'm disapproving and judgmental about my own flaws and inadequacies. (R)	☐ 5	☐ 4	☐ 3	☐ 2	☐ 1
12	I'm intolerant and impatient towards those aspects of my personality I don't like. (R)	☐ 5	☐ 4	☐ 3	☐ 2	☐ 1

Now tally your score and divide your total by 12 to determine your mean score.

Average overall self-compassion scores tend to be around 3.0 on the scale, so you can interpret your overall score accordingly. Scores between 1 and 2.5 reflect low self-compassion, whereas scores between 2.5 and 3.5 reflect moderate self-compassion.

Journal Reflection:

Was your score what you expected? When you make mistakes, fail in some way, or struggle with difficulties, how do you generally talk to yourself? Do you criticize and attack yourself or do you self-soothe with compassionate understanding?

Consider re-taking the self-compassion scale when you finish reading this book to see if your level of self-compassion has changed.

Defining Self-Compassion

Self-compassion is *maître* in Sanskrit, which means unconditional friendliness with and positive regard for the self. In Hebrew, self-compassion translates as "merciful, steadfast love." According to Dr. Neff, self-compassion consists of three things:[45]

- *Self-kindness.* Relating warmly and kindly to ourselves, rather than being self-critical whenever we're faced with our own shortcomings or encounter difficulties
- *Common humanity.* Remembering that suffering and failure are part of our shared human experience rather than unique to us as individuals
- *Mindfulness.* Meeting our difficult feelings in a balanced way so we don't over-identify with them

Benefits of Self-Compassion

Through regular practice, you can develop self-compassion. In fact, it need not take long at all. Following any painful experience where you trip up or "get it wrong," self-compassion can help to defuse your difficult feelings.

After only a short time practicing, you will be able to nurture a greater sense of well-being and emotional control and respond compassionately to others. You will be better able to accept that it is a common human experience to make mistakes—and you don't have to beat yourself up when it happens.

Research has shown that practicing self-compassion improves well-being, life satisfaction, resilience, and sense of connection with others.[46] At the same time, self-compassion prevents the downward spiral created by self-criticism, rumination, and shame so that you can recover faster after failing in some way or making a mistake.

As Neff's pioneering work has shown, self-compassion is a skill that can be learned. Neff developed the eight-week Mindful Self-Compassion program to teach self-compassion skills. Working with Chris Germer, her colleague at Harvard University, Neff conducted a randomized controlled trial in 2013. Results demonstrated that self-compassion practice can have a dramatic effect on one's natural sense of self-compassion. Neff's MSC program increased participants' self-compassion levels by 40% in one year.[47] When you think about it, those results are impressive, and no doubt we can all benefit from raising our self-compassion levels.

Self-compassion helps you recognize and soothe your painful thoughts and emotions with understanding and acceptance, and with practice, this gets easier. Which parts of your character make you blush or lose your temper? By regularly practicing self-compassion, you can stop berating yourself for what you perceive to be your flaws and shortcomings. Instead, you can approach them with the same understanding you would show to a colleague who possesses the same traits.

Like every other human being on the planet, you are imperfect. You make mistakes. When things don't go as you intended, try not to shrink away from others or feel isolated in your imperfection. Remember: the world is filled with imperfect yet beautiful human beings.

Everybody has a bad day now and then. You can learn how to be gentle with yourself when things go wrong or when you make mistakes so that you feel less vulnerable.

Building Self-Compassion

A moment of self-compassion can change your entire day.
A string of such moments can change the course of your life.

—Christopher Germer

When we bring self-compassion into everyday life, we learn to be kind to ourselves. The first step in becoming more self-compassionate is to notice when you are being self-critical or reactive. Your body reacts when you are self-critical. When you catch yourself in the act of finding fault with yourself, shift your attention instead to your body. You might notice your shallow breathing, warm face, or clenched belly.

Once you become aware of reactivity, you can set the intention to release it—letting go of the bodily tension and hostile thoughts and extending kindness to yourself instead.

You can quickly become familiar with practices designed to build your self-compassion. Below are a couple of suggestions from Neff's website.[48]

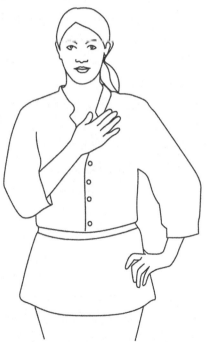

Take a Self-Compassion Break

Practice mindful self-compassion when things aren't going the way you want them to. Maybe you're late for work or have just had an argument with a colleague. Rather than getting caught up in reactivity, take a self-compassion break.

Try This:
Self-Compassion Break

As a way of connecting with the difficult experience you are in or just went through, make a comforting physical gesture to yourself (example: placing your hand over your heart). Sense yourself opening up to compassion, and send kindness to the hurt inside. Kindness in the form of physical gestures can have a soothing effect on your body. It doesn't matter what the gesture is, as long as it resonates with you and you find it comforting. According to Neff, such gestures activate the parasympathetic system and have a calming effect, helping you to unhook from the storyline of painful thoughts and feelings.

Speak kindly to yourself. When you find yourself in the grip of strong feelings of distress or self-judgment, you may find yourself thinking, "I'm hopeless" or other condemning comments. However, thinking like this only makes you feel worse. Instead, substitute kind phrases to help calm your distress. Choose phrases that resonate with you, such as these that Neff suggests, and memorize them, repeating them silently whenever you need compassion.

- *This is a moment of suffering.* (Here, mindfulness helps you acknowledge what is happening.)
- *Suffering is part of life.* (This helps you to remember your common humanity; you are by no means alone in your suffering.)
- *May I be kind to myself in this moment.* (This phrase helps you respond compassionately rather than berate yourself.)

Do you feel soothed and comforted after taking a self-compassion break? If not, don't worry, as this practice can feel a little awkward at first. Be patient. It may take time and practice to feel at ease extending kindness to yourself.

Try This:
Compassionate Letter Writing

Bring to mind an issue you have that makes you feel bad about yourself—perhaps relating to your appearance or a mistake you made that still rankles. Now, see in your mind's eye a friend who is unconditionally compassionate and wise and try to adopt the perspective of that person, seeing yourself through their eyes. Imagine that this friend can see all your strengths and weaknesses, including what you dislike about yourself.

Ask yourself what this friend would say to you right now, from their compassionate perspective, about your issue. Sit down and write a letter to yourself as though it were from your friend, focusing on the issue that's troubling you.

Once you finish, put the letter aside for a while. Then come back and read it later, allowing the words to really sink in.

Journal Reflection:

Following this practice, take a moment to reflect.

How did you find this self-compassion practice?

How was it for you to change from negative, self-berating thoughts to extending kind, compassionate words to yourself?

Did you feel soothed and comforted by these compassionate sentiments?

Self-Compassion Is Healthy

The ability to be self-compassionate is closely linked to the ability to be compassionate toward others. If you are self-compassionate, you are better able to practice healthy self-care. Given the nature of your work, it is crucial for you to develop self-compassion to help prevent compassion fatigue, and to effectively provide compassionate care to others.

Self-compassion is a skill that anyone can (and should!) learn. Practicing it increases emotional strength and resilience, allowing a person to bounce back from difficult experiences and to overcome self-criticism. Self-compassion helps us acknowledge our shortcomings so we can accept and forgive ourselves, making whatever changes are necessary, caring for ourselves and others in the best possible ways.

Practice Plan:

Take a self-compassion break at intervals throughout your day when things are difficult. Likewise, when you struggle to keep up your daily practice, be kind and encourage yourself rather than beat up on yourself.

As best you can, keep up your formal daily practice by alternating sitting meditation with mindful movement and walking meditation. Continue to bring mindful awareness to your daily activities.

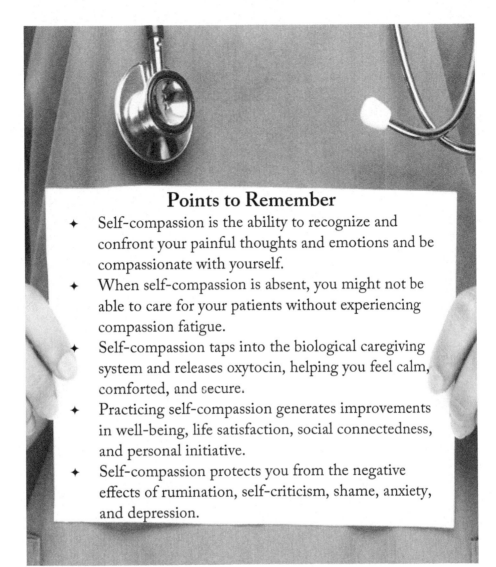

Points to Remember

+ Self-compassion is the ability to recognize and confront your painful thoughts and emotions and be compassionate with yourself.

+ When self-compassion is absent, you might not be able to care for your patients without experiencing compassion fatigue.

+ Self-compassion taps into the biological caregiving system and releases oxytocin, helping you feel calm, comforted, and secure.

+ Practicing self-compassion generates improvements in well-being, life satisfaction, social connectedness, and personal initiative.

+ Self-compassion protects you from the negative effects of rumination, self-criticism, shame, anxiety, and depression.

CHAPTER FOURTEEN

Strengthening Compassion

*Many of us think that compassion drains us, but I promise you
it is something that truly enlivens us.*

—Joan Halifax

Think back to the self-compassion quiz you took in Chapter 13. Are you kind to yourself? Whatever your score, don't worry. That's simply your own personal starting block. Compassion levels are never set in stone. Ultimately, compassion is a skill, and just as you trained to be a nurse, you can train to be compassionate. For many, compassion comes more quickly and easily than nursing training—and increases with practice.

Compassion isn't exclusive, a talent reserved only for certain people. Just like a weak muscle, compassion strengthens with training. Almost anyone can learn to be more compassionate and kinder with themselves and others.

Melinda, a nurse who worked on an ICU step-down floor, discovered this for herself. Her many patients were all very sick, requiring a great deal of care. Melinda felt stressed and regularly argued with coworkers who seemed unwilling to lend a hand. While she ran from room to room, she could not hide her contempt for anyone who did not give 110% to their work as she did. One day her anger boiled over when she perceived a colleague slacking. She decided to confront him at his desk, in front of everyone, which accomplished nothing—except now Melinda's coworkers avoided her, adding to her stress.

One of Melinda's close nursing friends worked on a different floor, and they would meet regularly for coffee. Her friend listened kindly to Melinda's never-ending frustrations and then smiled. The hospital was hosting a nine-week compassion training, open to all. At first Melinda flatly refused to go, but her friend finally talked her into giving it a go.

As the compassion training progressed, Melinda realized that many of her feelings were signs of not taking care of herself. She learned how to be kinder to herself, manage her anger, and clearly and compassionately address her issues with colleagues. By reminding herself to be compassionate first toward herself, she was able to handle her negative feelings. As she realized that they were all in this together and that it was difficult for everyone, she was more able to be compassionate toward her patients and colleagues—even the difficult ones.

Although Melinda's natural capacity for compassion may be what drew her to nursing, work-related stress and time pressures compromised her ability to fully express this innate characteristic. Unfortunately, that can happen to you, as well. In order to thrive, your compassionate instinct needs your time and care, your nurturing cultivation. You need to set the intention to actively cultivate compassion in your everyday life, especially when you work in a stressful environment where you are overly busy and resources are scarce.

Consider This:

How often do you argue with coworkers during a shift? Do you sit alone during breaks or meal times? How often have you passed someone in the hall and said to yourself a hurtful comment like, "Fat slob" or "Talk about a bad hair day"? How often have you sat at the nursing station and complained about a particular patient's behavior?

Innovative compassion practices drawn from contemplative two-thousand-year-old meditation traditions can help strengthen your compassion. Studies on the results of these practices, which are now being taught in cities across the globe, show that the brain is malleable, like muscles. Such programs help individuals learn to cope with stress, be more present, and exhibit more compassion at work and in everyday life.

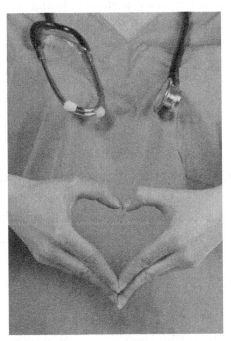

Loving-Kindness

One of the best-known compassion practices is loving-kindness: the cultivation of goodwill or kindheartedness. Besides culturing the heart, loving-kindness is also a practice for wishing oneself and others well. It helps you to redirect your attention away from negative thoughts to what you most want for others and yourself. Through loving-kindness, you connect with a genuine wish for happiness for all beings.

This ancient and beautiful practice helps you to treat others and yourself with greater kindness. It helps dissolve harsh, critical sentiments and creates an environment in your heart for love, empathy, and goodwill to grow. With practice, you are released from resentment, suffering, and are free to extend goodwill to others and to yourself.

As a mindfulness teacher, when I teach loving-kindness practice to healthcare professionals, I am always moved by their responses, even during short moments of practice spanning fifteen minutes or less. Many participants visibly relax and soften. Some weep. Connection between group members invariably deepens.

Try This:
Loving-Kindness Meditation

The following is a guided loving-kindness meditation. You can do this practice sitting down or lying on a bed or mat. If you can only do short segments of the full practice, that's fine. Start slowly and move through it at your own pace. (To access a guided audio recording of this practice, visit www.nursingmindfully.com.)

Let your eyes close or leave them slightly open, casting your gaze toward the floor. Feel your breath in your belly, chest, or nostrils—wherever it feels most prominent—letting your awareness rest there for a while.

When you feel settled, gradually move your awareness to your heart and chest, allowing this region to soften, letting go of tension with each exhale.

Allow an image of yourself to arise, as though you can see yourself standing right in front of you. Connecting with the energy of warmth in your heart, begin extending kind wishes toward yourself. You might wish yourself health, happiness, or serenity. Make these wishes concrete by generating phrases that give them expression:

(cont'd)

May I be healthy.
May I be peaceful.
May I be happy.

Focus on the phrases that feel most important to you, repeating them to yourself, feeling your heart envelop the words as they generate a feeling of kindness toward yourself.

If you don't feel the kindness, or the practice doesn't come naturally to you, don't worry. Many people find it difficult to be kind to themselves. Just keep focusing gently on your intention, even if the feeling isn't there, repeating the phrases softly, feeling their essence.

After you send loving-kindness to yourself, bring to mind someone who has helped or extended kindness to you, perhaps a mentor or teacher. Imagine this person in front of you, and wish them well:

May you be healthy.
May you be peaceful.
May you be happy.

If thoughts come up as you do this, just notice them without judgment and come back to repeating the phrases.

Next, picture a close friend or family member, wishing them well in the same way with the same thoughts and phrases.

Now bring to mind a person you see occasionally but do not know well. It could be someone who serves you at the café or gas station. You may feel indifferent toward this person and may not even know their name. Still, wish them well in the same way, using the same kind thoughts and phrases.

Now call to mind a person you find difficult: someone with whom you've had some conflict. Go slowly. Choose someone

(cont'd)

with whom the conflict (or your level of affect) is minor. (It's best at the outset not to pick someone you have intense feelings toward as you may feel overwhelmed.) Begin by wishing them well in the same fashion as you did with the previous persons, repeating the same good wishes and phrases. If you get distracted or lost in thought, that's okay. Just steer yourself gently back, silently repeating one kind phrase at a time and directing it toward that person.

Now, release this person from your mind's eye and mentally bring all four people in front of you, noticing how it feels to wish yourself and all of them well.

Try expanding this further, sending loving-kindness beyond your small circle— to strangers, to people everywhere, to animals and insects, to trees and plants, feeling your goodwill expand without limits.

Gradually bring your attention back to your breath, slowly opening your eyes.

Journal Reflection:
What did you notice during this practice?
> How was it to send loving-kindness to a difficult person?
> How do you feel after doing this practice?

Loving-Kindness Practice for Nurses

Sharon Salzberg, one of the world's foremost meditation teachers and author of *Loving-Kindness: The Revolutionary Art of Happiness*, has offered the following loving-kindness practice specifically for caregivers.[49] (The phrases in this meditation may resonate with you, helping you to offer kindness without being attached to the outcome, especially when the outcome is beyond your control. Given the work you do, this can often be the case.)

Try This:
Loving-Kindness Practice for Caregivers

Settle into a comfortable sitting posture, gently closing your eyes. Allow your back to be straight but not stiff. As you take a few deep breaths, notice your body relaxing, and your chest softening. When you feel ready, silently repeat the following phrases to yourself:

May I find the inner resources to be able to give to others and to receive myself.

May I remain peaceful and let go of expectations.

May I offer love, knowing I can't control the course of life, suffering, or death.

I care about your pain, yet I know I cannot control it.

I wish you happiness and peace but cannot make your choices for you.

May I recognize my limits compassionately, just as I recognize the limitations of others.

As you repeat the phrases, feel the meaning of the words, letting them sink deeply into your heart.

Compassion, often the ultimate gift of nurse to patient, must be nourished to be sustained.

— *Compassion Fatigue and Burnout in Nurses Who Work with Children with Chronic Conditions and Their Families,* by Jennifer Maytum, Mary Heiman, and Ann Garwick

Short Moments of Practice Matter

Loving-kindness meditation generates a sense of a "warm glow" around others—you may experience the person to whom you extend loving-kindness as familiar, similar, and connected to you. This warm glow helps you develop compassion for everyone—including difficult colleagues and challenging patients.

Loving-kindness is a time- and cost-effective practice. Even brief sessions have been shown to be beneficial. Just ten minutes of practice can increase your feelings of connection and closeness to others.[50] This is good news for busy nurses on tight schedules.

Need another incentive? Loving-kindness practice may also keep the aging process at bay. This has been confirmed by research that shows telomere length is relatively longer in women who practice loving-kindness.[51] (Telomeres are small bits of chromosomes whose length is shortened by the negative effects of stress.) Maybe it's time to let go of your anti-aging products and practice loving-kindness instead!

Loving-Kindness for Back Pain

Did you know that loving-kindness meditation can help reduce pain, anger, and psychological distress in people with persistent low back pain?

Larry Wall, a nurse who worked at the local hospital's Alzheimer unit, discovered first-hand the benefits of loving-kindness. Larry loved and cared for his patients the best he could, although the nature of the work led to frustration at times. His patients often had episodes of agitation and aggression, and continuously wandered into other patients' rooms. Still, Larry was well able to keep his feelings of frustration under control.

One of his favorite patients, Pearl, was on a downhill slide. As the late afternoon light faded to sundown, Pearl regularly suffered sensory confusion. She would see the trees outside as intruders and would become aggressive and paranoid. Her paranoia increased as time wore on, and, finally, she began to see the CNA who helped with her self-care activities as an attacker. One evening, Pearl tripped and fell to the floor as she fought off the startled CNA who was helping her get ready for bed. Staff were called to help her up and bring her to bed. As Larry tried to lift her, Pearl wrestled free, and suddenly Larry felt a sharp pain in his lower back.

When Larry woke the next morning, his back was tight and in spasm. After unsuccessful visits to several doctors, he finally went to a surgeon who operated on his herniated disc, but sadly, the operation didn't take away the pain. Larry walked around in pain most days and was unable to return to work as planned.

He tried massage, chiropractic, and physical therapy, and although these provided temporary relief, they didn't help in the long term. One day, while he was lying on the couch trying to cope with a particularly bad bout of pain, Larry saw a TV show about a loving-kindness program at Stanford University. He had always been open to meditation, and he put the practice to immediate use, sending himself loving-kindness right there and then, as he struggled with unpleasant sensations. Instead of getting caught up in a story about how long the pain might last, he focused instead on extending loving-kindness to himself in that moment of suffering. Eventually, after practicing loving-kindness over many days, sometimes twice a day, Larry found that his back didn't hurt as much. The loving kindness "medication" became a natural daily ritual. After six months off work, Larry returned to his unit, where his loving-kindness practice sustained him through the daily challenges he encountered.

Research supports Larry's experience of the healing effects of loving-kindness meditation on back pain. James Carson and his colleagues at the Duke University Medical Center tested an eight-week loving-kindness program on patients with chronic low-back pain.[52] Patients were randomly assigned to one of two groups: one that was taught the practice of loving-kindness or one that received standard care. Throughout the program, the pain, anger, and psychological distress of all patients in the study were assessed.

The loving-kindness group reduced their pain and psychological distress levels—whereas the standard-care group did not improve. Interestingly, the benefits of loving-kindness were "dose-related." An analysis of the patients' diaries showed that when they practiced more loving-kindness on a given day, they experienced less pain that day— as well as less anger the following day. [53] Even after the study ended, the loving-kindness group retained their benefits.

Documented evidence shows that loving-kindness helps reduce everything from migraines, stress, and the risk of cardiovascular disease to anxiety and negative emotions,[54] but the benefits don't stop there. The practice also helps balance blood pressure, promote positive emotions, and improve brain function.

All of this benefits everyday lives, especially those of nurses. Nursing work is stressful—physically and emotionally demanding. The daily grind can cause back issues, ill health, and emotional distress. Fortunately, loving-kindness meditation can help counteract these difficulties.

Cultivating Compassion

While loving-kindness is the wish for the happiness and welfare of others, compassion is the feeling that arises when you encounter suffering and feel motivated to relieve it. When you wish someone happiness, you are practicing loving-kindness, and when someone is suffering and you feel compelled to try to reduce their suffering, you are practicing compassion. Although the qualities of loving-kindness and compassion are related, compassion is the more challenging of the two because it arises when you witness and empathize with another's pain.

It is very wonderful to sit close to someone
who has compassion in his or her heart.
—Thich Nhat Hanh

Just Like Me

You can practice compassion in different ways and in various contexts. It's useful in situations in which you struggle to understand and empathize with other people's perspectives. If you have difficulty connecting with a colleague, patient, or someone else in your life, you can try a practice called "Just Like Me." When you're able to perceive that person as similar to yourself (just like me), you may be more able to feel and behave positively toward them. When you spend time and effort creating thoughts of similarity to others, this way of thinking and feeling becomes habitual over time, and your relationships benefit.

Try This:
Just Like Me

Sit in a relaxed yet alert state, and close your eyes. Take a few deep breaths, allowing the in-breath and out-breath to be long and slow, as drawn-out as you can comfortably manage.

Bring the person you are having difficulty with to mind.

As you picture them, notice how you feel in your body and mind, especially any changes or increased tension.

Take a moment to reflect on the truth that, just like you, this person is a human being. Keeping this in mind, silently and slowly repeat the following:

This person wishes happiness in life, just like me.

This person has at some time in life been lonely, sad, and confused, just like me.

(cont'd)

223

This person has made mistakes and has regrets, just like me.
This person wishes to be free from suffering, just like me.
This person wishes to be loved and appreciated, just like me.

When you can truly empathize with this person, the understanding grows that they, too, suffer and feel the same kinds of pain you do.

As you feel your heart soften and open to this person, do you feel a desire that they be free from suffering? If so, stay with that feeling and notice how it is expressed in your body. Allow the feeling to grow while your heart opens further.

You can now connect with some positive wishes for this person:
May this person be free from suffering.
May this person learn to cope wisely with life's challenges.
May this person be happy.
Because this person is a human being. Just like me.

Gradually direct your focus back to your breathing, gently opening your eyes and bringing your attention into the room.

Journal Reflection:

Take a few moments to notice if you feel any differently now than before you did this practice.

What, if anything, did you experience as difficult?

What did you discover?

Compassion practice helps to remind you that others are human, too. As a result, they make mistakes, just as you do. They also feel pain, suffering, and rejection, just like you. With practice, you may find that compassion arises quite naturally and readily during your day and that regular practice uproots negative thoughts and emotions you might be harboring. When you remember that all people share a common humanity, you can more easily shift gears and change your perspective. With practice, resentment and hostility are replaced with a sense of connectedness while a natural compassion for others and yourself grows.

Nurse Phil Peterson, who worked on a neurological unit in the local hospital, told me about his experience. Although Phil respected his manager, he could not seem to get along with her. She would constantly minimize the work he did, even though he was excellent at his job. Oftentimes, she would call him into the office and reprimand him for his faults and failings. She accused him of taking too much time to get pain pills for patients and insisted his assessment of complex neuro patients wasn't up to the required standard. Whenever Phil saw her doing rounds in the unit, his breath would catch in his throat and his heart would pound.

Fortunately, Phil was a meditator who regularly attended retreats. To help him deal with his overbearing manager, he knew he had to put his meditation into practice. He began to practice a daily compassion meditation during which he focused on her. Over time, as he brought the supervisor to mind, he began to realize how much responsibility she carried as head of the neuro unit. She was under tremendous stress as she fulfilled the demands of her role. His manager was *just like him.* Gradually, as his heart began to soften toward her, he was able to wish her well in his meditations.

While Phil had previously avoided his manager at every opportunity, after some weeks of compassion practice, he was able to approach her. As she scrutinized his practice and patient care during his shift, he took a moment to become grounded, compassionately recognizing the fear in her eyes. After responding that he had no incidents to report, he took a deep breath and asked, "How are you this morning? I notice you look tense. Is there anything I can do to help?"

Phil held his breath, expecting a tirade, but his manager looked at him and said, "You know, you are the only person on this unit who has ever asked how I am and offered to help. Thank you for that."

Although his manager continued to show signs of stress, and was still occasionally critical, Phil had an understanding of how she felt. He maintained his compassion for her struggles and forgave her for taking her stress out on him. The reality was that he wasn't afraid of her anymore. When he saw her walking around the unit, his heart felt open and friendly toward her as he remembered that, *just like him*, she was doing the best she could under difficult circumstances.

Tonglen-on-the-Spot

Tonglen is another practice for activating compassion. A Tibetan word, *tonglen* means, "taking in and sending out." In tonglen, you take in the pain and suffering of others (and of yourself) and send out relief, compassion, and happiness. Tonglen helps counter the tendency to resist emotional discomfort. Rather than pushing away pain, tonglen invites us to move toward it. Although it seems counterintuitive to do this, tonglen is a profound and effective practice for cultivating compassion for ourselves and others.

Formal tonglen practice can be rather complicated for those who are new to it. While formal tonglen might be more than you are ready for at present, you can still practice what is known as "tonglen-on-the-spot." Essentially, with your in-breath, you consciously take in the suffering you see around you. On the out-breath, you willingly send out relief, kindness, and well-being.

You can practice tonglen-on-the-spot in everyday situations. Undoubtedly, on the hospital floor or in your office, there are countless times each day when you encounter challenging and difficult situations. Start with the practice as it is described below. Then, as you go about your day, pause and practice it whenever you come face-to-face with someone who is suffering. Breathe in any pain that you encounter. As you breathe out, focus on sending the person your peace, joy, and contentment.

Try This:
Tonglen-on-the-Spot

Bring to mind a patient who is in mental or physical pain. See yourself sitting calmly with this person, holding their image and energy clearly, as you breathe slowly in and out.

Now, let yourself breathe in this person's pain, allowing it to penetrate your heart.

With the exhale, release the pain, while sending the person all the contentment you have known in your lifetime.

Journal Reflection:

When you finish practicing tonglen-on-the-spot, reflect on your experience.

Did this practice come naturally to you or did you struggle with it?

As you reflect on your experience now, how do you feel?

As you learn to approach and stay with discomfort, your compassion will grow, and you will be more able to connect with those who are suffering, quite naturally breathing in that person's pain and sending out happiness. That's tonglen-on-the-spot.

You can also practice this when strong emotions come up at work and you feel stressed or confused by coworkers. Perhaps you experience conflict with a coworker or supervisor and things become heated. Then angry words are exchanged. Instead of reacting, take a pause to practice tonglen-on-the-spot, breathing in the discord and difficult feelings. On the out-breath, have a sense of silently extending warmth and ease to both yourself and the other person.

Later you might choose to address the conflict directly with the person. Taking the time to practice tonglen-on-the-spot first may help you respond in a clear and more balanced way.

A person who has awakened the force of genuine compassion will be quite capable of working physically, verbally, and mentally for the welfare of others.

—Jamgon Kongtrul

June Boyle is a holistic nurse who works in cancer care. A cancer survivor herself, she is a long-time meditator. She attends a weeklong meditation retreat annually, and this sustains her in her challenging work. On the hospital floor or in her office, she encounters difficult situations countless times a day.

As she goes about her work, June pauses and practices tonglen-on-the-spot whenever she has discord with a colleague or when she comes face-to-face with someone who is suffering. When a patient is in distress, she breathes in the pain she encounters. As she breathes out, she sends the person her peace, joy, and contentment. Tonglen-on-the-spot is a practice you can draw on privately, at a moment's notice, as June does, to sustain you in your work.

Daily Loving-Kindness and Compassion

Don't limit loving-kindness and compassion meditation to formal practices removed from your everyday life. Each day, set an intention to bring your goodwill and kind heart into your relationships at work and at home. Practice loving-kindness and compassion by sending warmth, friendliness, and goodwill to everyone with whom you come in contact. Practice with family, friends, and colleagues, as well as the patients in your care—including the difficult ones. Notice how good it feels to extend loving-kindness and compassion.

Val Heraty, an ER nurse in a busy urban hospital, sets the intention to practice compassion every day at work. Introduced to meditation by her parents at a young age, Val feels well-resourced to handle the stresses that come with the job. Every morning she wakes up early to have time for meditation. Her first thought of the morning is a *gatha*, a verse that helps her set a compassionate intention for the day. She repeats the *gatha* phrase, following her breath in and out, and once she completes her meditation, she gets out of bed and starts her day.

Try This:
Compassion Mantra

As you awaken each morning, try repeating a *gatha*, a simple phrase to help you focus your intention to be compassionate this day.

The following is a *gatha* which dharma teacher Poep Sa Frank Jude Boccio adapted from Thich Nhat Hanh.[55] If it resonates with you, recite it upon waking, or compose your own:

Waking this morning, I smile.
A brand new day is before me.
I aspire to live each moment mindfully,
And to look upon all beings
With the eyes of kindness and compassion.

This next exercise can help you develop the habit of using tonglen and the other practices learned in this section.

Try This:
Compassion Reflection

Before going to sleep each evening, take time to reflect on how compassionate you were with the people you met this day. Jot down your thoughts if writing helps you with the reflection process. Simply contemplate the day's events and how you responded to them, without judging yourself harshly.

Reflect on these questions:

How well did you do?

When did you act with compassion?

Where were you blocked?

Can you see why you were compassionate in one situation but not in another?

In what ways could you have done better?

What did you learn?

Compassionate Leadership

Although this chapter outlines ways in which formal practices can strengthen your innate compassion, it is important to remember that compassion can be strengthened in other ways, too. On-the-job training, workshops, classes, and online resources all offer possibilities for growing compassion.

The Journal of Nursing Management published a twelve-year study of nurses who attended compassionate-care training.[56] Initially, all the student nurses learned how to be compassionate in their work. However, when the new nurses started shadowing a senior nurse as part of their training, the student nurses assigned to an uncompassionate senior nurse failed to continue their compassionate behavior, while the ones who had a compassionate senior nurse continued to show compassion.

The implications of these findings are clear. Senior nurses play a key role in helping student nurses become compassionate caregivers. If you are a senior nurse, remember to be the best compassion role model you can be when you work with nurses in training.

At work or at home, you can strengthen the muscles of loving-kindness and compassion with the practices described in this chapter. Like mindfulness, loving-kindness and compassion are natural human qualities, and their cultivation requires time and practice.

You will find that, as you practice, your expanding levels of kindness and compassion will bring increasing amounts of calmness, peace, and contentment to your life and work, as well as to those around you.

Practice compassion patiently, moving at your own pace. Trust in the goodness of your heart and follow where it leads you.

Practice Plan:

Every day, alternate at least fifteen minutes of loving-kindness meditation or any of the compassion practices of your choice with mindfulness of breathing. If the formal practice is challenging, explore bringing loving-kindness into your day by silently extending kindness to someone that you meet or bring to mind.

Take a pause now in reading this book, so that you can integrate these practices fully before you move on to the final section.

Use your journal to reflect upon your experience so far with the various practices.

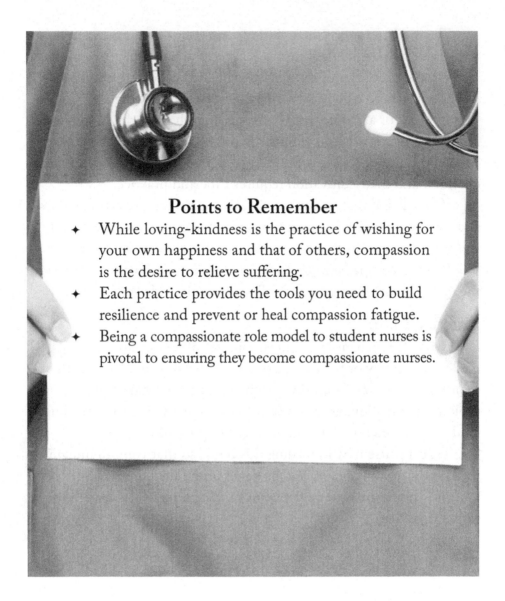

Points to Remember

✦ While loving-kindness is the practice of wishing for your own happiness and that of others, compassion is the desire to relieve suffering.

✦ Each practice provides the tools you need to build resilience and prevent or heal compassion fatigue.

✦ Being a compassionate role model to student nurses is pivotal to ensuring they become compassionate nurses.

PART IV
MINDFULNESS FOR BETTER PERFORMANCE

By letting it go, it all gets done. The world is won by those who let it go.
But when you try and try, the world is beyond winning.
—Lao Tzu

CHAPTER FIFTEEN

Working with Thoughts

Don't believe everything you think. Thoughts are just that—thoughts.
—Allan Lokos

Samantha was a certified nurse midwife who loved working with women throughout their pregnancies. However, she often felt anxious around doctors and other support personnel. Not everyone in the labor and delivery field respected her role as a midwife; some preferred obstetricians. In response, she was very sensitive to this issue. One night, while Samantha was working a case with a mom-to-be in labor, a coworker suggested she ask Dr. Smith for help. Samantha insisted she didn't need his help—she could take care of her patient herself.

Her mind began to race, though. While accompanying the patient through the process of giving birth, she couldn't keep her coworker's question out of her mind. She thought how rude it was for someone to suggest she needed help. She was every bit as good as Dr. Smith; in fact, she knew she brought a different, more personal level of care to her patients. It was insulting to suggest she needed help—she could easily handle this patient on her own. With her jaw clenched and a tension knot in her belly, Samantha continued to ruminate right throughout the baby's delivery. Normally, she would be fully absorbed in the whole process, but this time around, it was different. She was distracted and kept wondering about her coworker's comment and why anyone would think she needed help doing her job.

Have you ever been caught up in obsessive thinking the way Samantha was? When you are feeling a little low or stressed, do you take things to heart and replay or obsess over something you or someone else said or over something that happened?

This tendency to obsess in a negative way is known as *rumination*. It's the same word we use when a cow brings up food it has already eaten, to chew on all over again. That works for our farm friends, but doesn't work so well for us humans. Like a broken record, we rehash the scenario, but while the mind is trying to solve the problem, it actually creates a bigger one by intensifying our negative emotions. Negative thoughts affect our mood and stir up tension in the body, interfering with our ability to function well at work and at home. Meanwhile, we might waste hours overanalyzing the situation.

Thinking is a wonderful faculty—without it, you wouldn't be able to make sense of this book or make plans and decisions in your everyday life. But as we saw with Samantha, there is also a downside to thinking. Our thoughts are often negative and self-critical.

Consider This:

Have you ever jumped to conclusions over a comment made to you, or actions you observed from a distance? Do you look at constructive criticism as a slap in the face, or a stab in the back? When a nurse colleague suggests doing a task in a different way than yours, do you feel like you are being picked on? When you see other colleagues talking together, do you automatically feel they are talking about you?

Mindfulness of Thoughts

The primary cause of unhappiness is never the situation, but your thoughts about it. Be aware of the thoughts you are thinking.
—Eckhart Tolle

When you practice mindfulness, you are not trying to stop thinking. After all, thoughts are not seen as a problem. The thinking mind constantly generates thoughts; that is just what the mind does. Mindfulness helps you see your thoughts for what they are—fleeting images and sounds arising in the moment. You become consciously aware of them, with practice. When you are unaware of them, you can be driven *by* them, and when you automatically believe them to be true—as Samantha did—they can generate unhelpful reactions. Through mindfulness, you develop a different way of relating to your thoughts, in that you stop identifying with them and, instead, learn to let them be without getting trapped by them. With practice, you realize they are just thoughts and that you do not need to believe them or allow them to define you—and that they will pass. Imagine how knowing and understanding this basic truth would have changed Samantha's experience.

Take a moment right now to become aware of the thoughts arising in your mind. Just think: we have as many as seventy thousand thoughts a day, many of them a repeat of the thoughts we had yesterday!

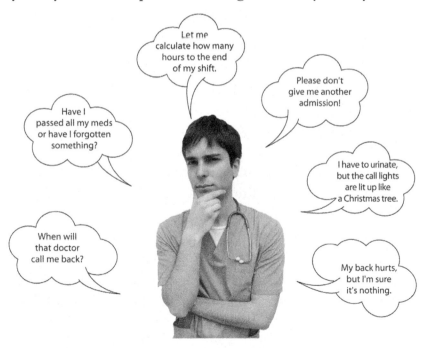

Observing Thoughts

The monkey mind is constantly generating thoughts, which may appear as images, sounds, fragments, judgments, or memories. Sometimes, these thoughts pass through us like clouds. At other times, we may identify with them and get hooked by them.

Mindfulness helps you notice when you are getting lost in thought. This helps you to unhook from the content of the thought so you can attend to what you are doing and what is going on around you. Let's say you are at a patient's bedside when you suddenly realize your attention is not with the patient but with what you have to do next. When you meet this thought with mindfulness, you can bring your attention back to your patient interaction. Each time you practice this, your mindfulness muscle grows stronger. Remember: learning to observe your thoughts in this way takes time and practice. To get started, you can try out this practice now.

Try This:
Observing Thoughts

Settle into a comfortable upright position. Gradually become aware of your breath, noticing the rhythm of the in-breath and out-breath.

In time, you may notice your attention is no longer with the breath but has wandered off into thinking.

Become aware of any thoughts that are present, accepting them without judgment. Thoughts are neither good nor bad.

Allow the thoughts to float like clouds in the sky, noticing each one as it arises, lingers for a while, and then dissolves.

There may be thoughts such as, "This is strange. I don't like this," or "This is interesting." Label the thoughts that arise with words such as "planning," "remembering," or "problem solving."

(cont'd)

Perhaps the thought passes as soon as you become aware of it and another thought follows.

Bring your attention back to the sensations of breathing until another thought pulls on your attention.

Notice what happens in your body while the thought is present. Is your neck tense? Is your chest heavy? Is your jaw clenched?

Bring an attitude of openness and curiosity to feelings and sensations. You may gently place your hand wherever you feel sensations in your body, and when they lessen, gently direct your focus back to the breath.

When you're ready to finish meditation, direct your attention to your breath and a sense of your whole body sitting and breathing. Then open your eyes and bring your attention into the room.

Journal Reflection:

What did you notice during this practice?

Were there a lot of thoughts or just a few compelling ones?

Did it take long to notice when your attention was swept away in the current of thinking?

When you focused on thoughts, did they dissipate? If so, that's not surprising. Many people experience thoughts dissolving once they become aware of them.

Some people relate to the metaphor of thoughts in the mind being like a waterfall. In the Observing Thoughts practice, mindfulness lets you step away from the current of the gushing water and observe from a distance the contents of your thoughts within the fall. This practice is quite similar to Mindfulness of Sounds which was introduced in Chapter 6. In the same way that sounds come and go, thoughts also come and go—and both trigger strong emotions that can easily hijack your attention.

In everyday life, you may often relate to your thoughts as if they were facts. We tend to see thoughts as facts because, if we think something, it feels as though the thought must therefore be true. With mindful attention, you realize that thoughts are just thoughts— mental processes in the mind—rather than the truth. From time to time, the current of the waterfall may sweep you in, but once you notice this, you can refocus, step back from your thoughts, and come into the present again. With practice, thoughts no longer bind you, and you recognize yourself as separate from your thoughts.

When you begin to understand how thoughts gain force in the mind, you have great freedom. The more you practice, the more you will be able to stay steady in the midst of life's ups and downs and the less likely you will be pulled into every scenario that unfolds in your mind.

It is remarkable how liberating it feels to be able to see that your thoughts are just thoughts and that they are not 'you' or 'reality.'
—Jon Kabat-Zinn

Marie was an LPN working in a small nursing home near her house. A widow with grown children, she lived alone—with only her thoughts for company. Although she kept busy, her thoughts so often preoccupied her that she couldn't make any real or meaningful contact with her colleagues and patients.

The list of things Marie worried about was endless: "Will my own health decline? If it does, how will I cope? Why didn't I spot my husband's illness sooner? Will I end up living out my days in a nursing home like this? How will my children cope without me? Will I live to see my grandchildren grow up? What if I start making mistakes at work and lose my job?" Marie's mind churned out worry after worry, and her days passed in a haze.

When Marie's daughter gave her a mindfulness course as a Christmas gift, she reluctantly enrolled. It was challenging for her even to sit still through the first few sessions. While Marie was always on the move in her everyday life, during these sessions, she had no distraction.

When Marie first practiced observing thoughts, her mind went wild with thoughts like, "I can't do this. This is not for me. I wish I hadn't come here. I can't feel my breath. This is not going to help." As her mind continued to spin out thoughts, Marie could barely contain herself.

However, she persisted and continued the practice at home. Slowly, things started to shift and her concentration gradually improved. The first change Marie noticed was that she could sit for several minutes focused on her breath. Then, when she had more stability, she could consciously direct her attention to her thoughts.

As the thoughts unfolded, she practiced seeing them as passing clouds, letting them run without paying much attention to them. Some thoughts were powerful and quickly gripped her. When this happened, she kindly brought her attention into her body. She labeled her feelings as fear, sadness, or some other emotion, and breathed with them. Then she returned her attention to her thoughts. For the first time in her life, Marie could sit and watch her thoughts with a kind attention, without being totally lost in them. It was profoundly freeing. Although there were still times the waterfall pulled her in, it felt like a weight had been lifted. She felt lighter and more at ease in her own skin.

Unhelpful Thinking Styles

A sick thought can devour the body's flesh more than fever or consumption.

—Guy de Maupassant

As you move through your workday, you may be unaware of the multitude of thoughts coursing through your mind. When there is a pattern to these thoughts, they are known as *unhelpful thinking styles*. Usually, they happen on autopilot outside your awareness and become deeply entrenched habits. Because your thoughts affect your emotions and bodily sensations, you may suddenly find your body tense or in the grip of anxiety or anger for no apparent reason. Once you know the most common unhelpful thinking styles, you will be more able to identify your own. From the descriptions below, can you identify your most common thinking patterns? What are your "Top Tunes?"

Jumping to Conclusions

- When you mind-read, you make assumptions about why something was said or done and conclude that it has to do with you.
  Examples:
  - The doctor on duty this morning yawned while I was talking to him. He must think I'm boring.
  - My patient was very reserved when I changed her bed linen. I wonder what I did wrong.

Magnification and Minimization

- When you magnify, you undermine yourself and magnify the positive attributes of others.
  Examples:
  - What if I give the wrong medicine to the patient and lose my license?
  - Why would anyone congratulate me on my patient care award when they know it's only a popularity contest?

Should/Shouldn't

- You set impossibly high standards for what you should be able to do and then you berate yourself when you can't reach these standards.

Examples:
- I know I shouldn't complain because I should be used to all this stress.
- I should go to work even when I'm sick so I don't let down my coworkers.

All-or-Nothing Thinking

You tend to see only one extreme or the other with no shades of gray in between.

Examples:
- If I can't cope on this unit. I should resign because I'm just not up to it.
- I made an error giving meds. I think it's time to give up nursing.

Mental Filter

You tend to have tunnel vision and focus on the negative aspects of a situation or yourself, while ignoring the positives.

Examples:
- Although we all worked well together to get through this shift, it doesn't change the fact that my coworkers are unreliable and it's always going to be this way.
- Even though I got the patient the help she needed, I missed that change in vital signs, so I failed as a nurse.

Personalization

You blame yourself or take responsibility for everything that goes (or could go) wrong, even though it's not your fault or responsibility.

Examples:
- I couldn't keep up with my assignments today because three nurses called in sick. I should still be able to keep up with everything.
- All the bad stuff happens to me when I'm on duty. Everyone else seems to get off easy.

Catastrophizing

🍃 You blow things out of proportion and assume something terrible is going to happen.
Examples:
- This one fall is going to get me fired. Since they don't go easy on nurses involved in falls, I know they are going to come down hard on me.
- I missed a medication dose overnight! Now the patient is going to get sick because of me, and my reputation will be ruined.

Overgeneralization

🍃 You use a negative aspect of the past or present to back up negative conclusions about current or future scenarios.
Examples:
- This facility is terrible because the charge nurse is always sitting on her butt at the station.
- She isn't a good nurse at all. Her call bells are always ringing, and she's never there to answer them.

Labeling

🍃 You assign negative labels to yourself and others.
Examples:
- She's not dependable, and would call in sick for a hangnail, leaving us to do her work.
- She thinks she's an expert who knows everything about medicine. Someone needs to tell her she's no more knowledgeable than the rest of us.

Emotional Reasoning

🍃 You base your view of yourself or situations on the way you feel rather than on facts.

Examples:

- I feel tired and frustrated. I'm just not cut out for working at the bedside.
- When it comes to patient care, I still feel like a failure, so I must be a failure.

Journal Reflection:

Take a moment now to reflect on the thinking styles and patterns you use most often.

How does thinking this way affect how you feel?

How does it affect your bodily sensations? (Do you clench, tighten, freeze, shake)?

How does thinking this way affect your work as a nurse?

Thoughts Are Just Thoughts

If you identify with some or all of these unhelpful thought styles, don't despair! From time to time, we all think in unhelpful ways. Mindfulness helps you shine the spotlight on negative thought patterns that have run rampant—and unchallenged—in your mind for years. Start to identify your patterns so you can loosen their grip on your life. Catch yourself in these negative patterns whenever you can. Remember, these thoughts are just that—thoughts, not facts. Then you can challenge the thought by asking yourself these questions:

What evidence do I have to support this thought?

Am I blaming myself for something that wasn't totally under my control?

Am I turning a molehill into a mountain (catastrophizing)?

Am I ignoring my strengths and focusing on my weaknesses?

What would I say to someone else if they told me this?

What would a friend or loved one say about this situation?

Challenging your thoughts with the questions above can release you from worries about what might go wrong in the future or from obsessing about what has already happened. Remember, you don't have to be a prisoner of your thoughts! Mindfulness opens the exit door. When you bring mindful awareness to your thoughts, you train your mind to settle and, with time and practice, realize you don't have to react to every passing thought. Instead, you can choose to let go of unhelpful thoughts that pop up in response to comments from coworkers or patients. Mindfulness puts you in charge of where you place your attention. Then, when you are less preoccupied with concerns and worries, you have more energy available to attend to your work. In addition, your peace of mind improves—and your patient care benefits, too!

Practice Plan:

Practice a short period of mindfulness of thoughts periodically this week and bring it into your daily routine. Also, set the intention to practice fifteen minutes of loving-kindness meditation daily. Continue bringing mindful awareness to your daily activities. Reflect on how your daily practice is progressing.

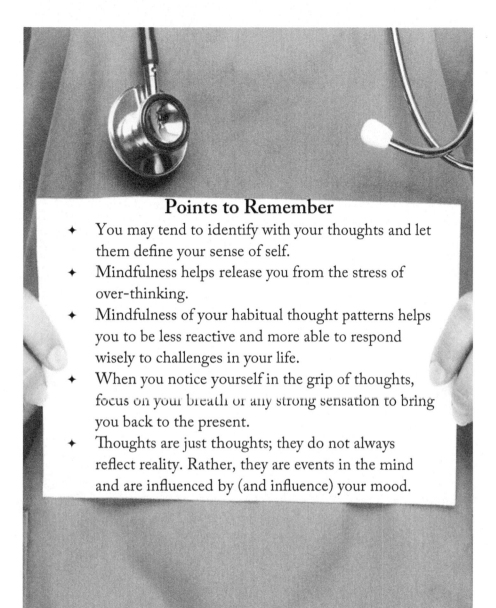

Points to Remember

+ You may tend to identify with your thoughts and let them define your sense of self.

+ Mindfulness helps release you from the stress of over-thinking.

+ Mindfulness of your habitual thought patterns helps you to be less reactive and more able to respond wisely to challenges in your life.

+ When you notice yourself in the grip of thoughts, focus on your breath or any strong sensation to bring you back to the present.

+ Thoughts are just thoughts; they do not always reflect reality. Rather, they are events in the mind and are influenced by (and influence) your mood.

CHAPTER SIXTEEN

Mindful Teamwork

When you come to work ready, happy, fresh, and at peace with
yourself, you help your coworkers to do the same. You go to work with
the aspiration of bringing peace, harmony, and well-being to your
coworkers and to the entire workplace.
You create happiness and harmony at work.
—Thich Nhat Hanh

One of the best things about being a nurse is how your job brings
you closer to others. The most worthwhile times of your career may
well be those special, shared moments between you and a patient
or colleague when you both experience the joy and connection of
working well together.

Synergy is the flow and harmony people experience by working
in sync with one another. A well-coordinated team works better
than one with members who are indifferent to or at odds with each
other. Undoubtedly, a group that is intelligent and dynamic enough
to respond to pressure in the environment *as a unit* can be more
productive and efficient. An on-the-ball company of nurses is like a
well-run ship or successful sports team: its sum is greater than its parts.

Colin Costello, a new nursing grad, discovered the importance
of teamwork while working his first week in the ICU unit. Colin was
overwhelmed by the gravity of his patients' illnesses and watched his
preceptor to learn what to do next. During one shift, a new trauma
patient arrived with a full list of orders.

All the nurses converged on the new arrival. Each person had a
place; they were experts in the tasks they took on. It made Colin feel

more relaxed about his new position knowing his coworkers on the unit could be counted on for help.

One nurse did vitals while another collected samples for routine screening. Colin was in charge of setting up the IV pump. While he did that, the respiratory therapist set up the ventilator. Each person took on a task, and before Colin realized it, the patient was set up, checked in, and ready for more specific care. The group of nurses didn't leave until all the admission orders were complete. Colin was impressed with how the nurses and technicians pulled together as a team. It helped make the critically ill patient as stable as possible and left the primary nurse free to begin paperwork for the new patient.

As with Colin's team, when your finely tuned team works together on the floor, the strong bonds you develop with each other mean that you never have to face anything alone. With the support of your colleagues, the inevitable trials and stresses of your nursing day are easier to manage. Likewise, your patients also benefit from an alert and harmonious team. Each member of your group has the satisfaction of knowing that even when they experience stress and tension, they do so within the context of a strong, supportive, and caring group.

Mindful Team Players

When nurses function as part of a unit, and when they act as part of a team, the job itself is easier and more efficient. Moreover, overall patient care is enhanced.

—Jennifer Ward

Just as a chain is only as strong as its weakest link, a group is only as strong as its weakest member. When you bring your own sense of presence to a group situation, you change the dynamic and encourage mindful presence within the group. Working together to achieve a focused goal means your group can achieve more than any single member can on their own. Successful group work results from a combination of self-awareness, awareness of others, and mindful attention to how the two dynamics interact.

Consider This:

Do you feel as though you are working alone, even though there may be five other nurses on the same ward as you? When you are unsure or having difficulties with a task, are you afraid or hesitant to ask another nurse for help? Have you ever misjudged a coworker's actions? Are you a gossip or complainer?

A group functioning with heightened awareness delivers more focused service to each patient. When the members of a group can respond well to challenges and difficulties, they offer something truly special to those under their care. Just as mindfulness can cultivate presence, resilience, calmness, and resourcefulness in an individual, it can do the same for the group. When all members are fully aware of their own processes and mindful of those of their colleagues, there is less miscommunication. It is easier to consciously choose behaviors that are more compassionate when the whole team is mindfully aware. An added benefit is that the energy saved through being mindful gives you more energy to bring to each patient.

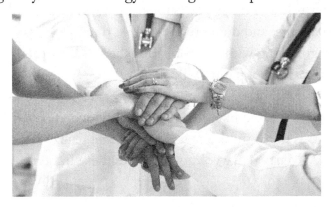

You may know people who complete the day's tasks—whether mundane or life-and-death emergencies—with the same calm and determined sense of responsibility. These people keep their heads when others around them are losing theirs. Not only do such people garner respect and admiration from their colleagues, they make others want to emulate them. If you make mindfulness a regular habit, you become a potential role model at work. When others notice the positive changes mindfulness practice creates for you, they may be encouraged to follow in your footsteps.

Alone we can do so little. Together we can do so much.

—Helen Keller

Conflict in Teams

Have you ever argued with someone and been surprised to find that their version of events is completely different from yours? Even though you shared the same experience, you each took away different things. Conflict often arises when you fail to examine what you think are obvious beliefs or when you make assumptions about others. Many times, conflict springs up because of misinterpretation or outright miscommunication.

Marty, a former mindfulness student of mine, told me how she learned this the hard way. Marty worked in a busy surgical practice. Her role as a nurse practitioner involved giving orders, admitting patients, and doing rounds while the doctor was in surgery. She usually got along with everyone, but she felt the other nurse practitioner in the group didn't like her.

Marty had seniority. Although the other nurse had only one year of experience, she acted like she knew it all, which annoyed Marty. "Who does this nurse think she is? Doesn't she realize I'm more experienced?" Marty replayed thoughts like these in her mind.

One day, Marty decided she had had enough and confronted the other nurse. They met in an empty patient room, and Marty expressed her concern about the animosity between them. Dismayed, the less-experienced nurse looked at Marty wide-eyed. She said she was simply doing her job and doing the best she could. She explained that she felt no animosity to anyone but that since she was relatively new to her role, she was trying to prove herself and compensate for her lack of confidence. Gradually, the truth of the situation dawned on Marty. She herself was the overbearing one, and the conflict that was playing out was in her own head. She left the meeting having realized that her own thinking, rather than the other nurse, was the problem.

When you are mindful, you anchor yourself in the present, and regularly check in with reality. Then you are less prone to being carried away with your *perceptions* of reality and all the baggage you bring with you. Unfortunately, Marty waited a long time to check in with reality; she let her assumptions and misinterpretations lead to conflict—at least in her mind.

In most cases of potential conflict, prevention is a better option than cure. Being mindful means that you are aware of difficulties as they occur and make smart, compassionate choices long before the situation has a chance to descend into conflict.

Knowing how to manage conflict is a vital skill for nurses. To this end, mindfulness is an important tool for good conflict resolution. It helps you know when to admit you're wrong, when to listen carefully, and how to move toward resolution and shared goals. Being open and attentive gives you the presence of mind to recognize if conflict is brewing, and the good sense to remedy it early.

Otherwise, you may run into problems if you waste mental resources on altercations with colleagues. Bullying, arguments, and disorganization take vital care and attention away from patients. The reality is you have way too much to do without being distracted by ongoing conflicts at work.

Even though you may not be the direct source of conflict or at the center of a disagreement, you can suffer by virtue of being part of a group in conflict. Procedures run less efficiently, everyone feels less satisfied, and threats may be posed to patient safety. Distracted or unhappy nurses carry that attitude over to their patients. Instead of modeling calm and compassion, they radiate stress and irritation.

Your Role in Your Team

Think about your work environment and your team. Who works toward group cohesion, encouraging healthy sharing, support, and goal-directed behavior? In particular, think of the people who have inspired you to do better work. In those moments when you felt proud to be part of a group effort, why do you think things worked so well, and what could you do now to recreate that spirit?

What role do you play on your team? Are you a cheerleader, a gossip, a lone wolf, or the one who chafes against rules and authority figures? Remember: your relationship to your workmates shapes the tone of the group. Who have you inspired? Who have you let down? Have there been times when you put your own grievances above the well-being of your patients?

Gossip

Catch yourself the next time you are gossiping about somebody; if you are aware of it, it will indicate an awful lot to you about yourself. Don't cover it up by saying that you are merely inquisitive about others. It indicates restlessness, a shallowness, a lack of real, profound interest in people.

—Jiddu Krishnamurti

What kind of conversations do you get into with coworkers? For example, do you talk behind people's backs? Do you gossip, condemn, scandalize, or complain? If so, notice how you feel during and after it. How does gossip impact your state of mind?

Trudy worked at a rural hospital where everyone knew everyone. She lived in the city and commuted to work, making her an outsider in a very insular community. The breakroom went quiet when she walked in. Many times, a nurse would find an excuse not to help her. Eventually, Trudy became aware that some nurses were gossiping about her. They said she was diverting pain medicines from patients, and some even questioned if she did any patient care, because she was always behind with her work. One nurse spread a rumor that Trudy was shamelessly flirting with the night phlebotomist. Since she was swamped all the time because she had no help, Trudy was frequently late getting out of the hospital. Meanwhile, she felt the animosity, and it was confirmed for her when her manager pulled her aside to see if any of the scathing gossip was true. It wasn't—and while telling him that was enough to put her manager's mind at ease, Trudy learned that she could not trust her coworkers. Their attitude created tension for her every shift she worked.

Gossip is toxic. If gossip is a persistent problem at work, then remember that your words have the power to curtail it. Speak out against nasty rumors when you encounter them and commit to being a voice of kindness and rationality in breakroom conversations.

If you indulge in idle talk, hearsay, or vicious attacks, then you take away attention and energy from your patients. Being mindful of your words means choosing not to participate in speech that harms. To decide whether your words qualify as harmful speech, imagine saying them directly to the person about whom you are talking. If you can't, then most likely they should not be voiced to others.

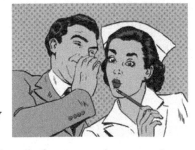

Try to use speech to build up—not break down—other people. Stick to the facts or excuse yourself from conversations that turn nasty. Most of all, be kind. Take care to cultivate harmonious and nourishing interactions with your coworkers and bring harmony and synergy to your workplace.

> ## Try This:
> ### Mindful Speech
> Ask yourself these questions:
>> Do my actions and words align with my higher purpose?
>> Whom do I admire, and how can I become more like them?
>> What is the effect of my attitude on those around me?

Becoming mindful of your speech patterns helps you to respond to others with an open heart and mind. As humans—and as conscious, responsible, and mindful members of any group—we always have room for improvement. With mindful attention to your interactions with colleagues, you can bring positive changes to your workplace, resulting in benefits for everyone, including yourself.

Practice Plan:

Observe your interactions with your coworkers this week. What are your strengths? Where do you fall short? Notice any judgments you hold about particular people, and be aware of any impulse to gossip or criticize. Then notice what it feels like to abstain and say nothing. In moments of conflict, practice Tonglen-on-the-Spot or Just Like Me. Continue to alternate or combine the formal practices you have learned so far in whatever combinations you choose.

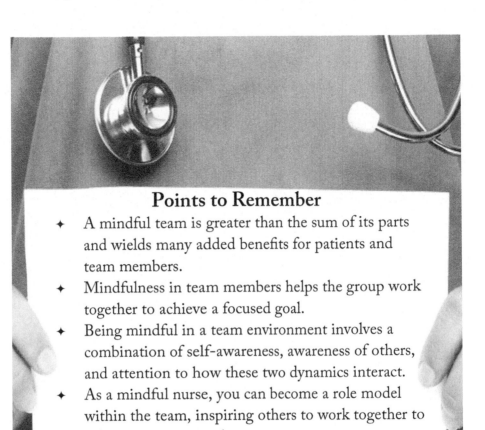

Points to Remember

+ A mindful team is greater than the sum of its parts and wields many added benefits for patients and team members.
+ Mindfulness in team members helps the group work together to achieve a focused goal.
+ Being mindful in a team environment involves a combination of self-awareness, awareness of others, and attention to how these two dynamics interact.
+ As a mindful nurse, you can become a role model within the team, inspiring others to work together to achieve common goals.
+ Each mindful team member encourages cooperation and mutual support and provides a safe environment for conflict resolution.

CHAPTER SEVENTEEN
Mindful Communication

I vow to cultivate loving speech and deep listening in order to bring joy and happiness to others and to relieve them of their suffering.
—Thich Nhat Hanh

Julie Carroll is a new nurse in a mental health unit. Although she enjoyed talking with her patients and getting to know them, she found it difficult and unsettling to engage with the more challenging patients. Her coworker Ger seemed to have a special way of talking to even the most agitated patients.

When a patient went on a rampage and destroyed the crafts room, Julie wanted to medicate her. Ger objected and insisted on talking with the patient instead. He gently calmed her down by listening to what was bothering her. In the end, the patient felt heard. She settled down and didn't need to be medicated.

Of course, Julie wanted to know how Ger did that. To explain, he described how important it is to be fully present when interacting with others, especially those who are distressed. Ger related how, in difficult situations, he first checks in with himself—he pauses and takes a breath or two to center himself and avoid coming from a reactive place. When he gets distracted, he brings his attention back to the situation at hand.

In this instance, he sat with the patient and let her talk openly about her feelings and air her grievances. Importantly, he let go of judgments about how she acted out and created havoc, and talked to her in a way that allowed her to open up and express her frustration. In other words, he stayed calm and let the patient lead. With coworkers, he interacts the same way. Instead of becoming offended when things get heated, he asks questions about the source of the disagreement until everyone can come to an understanding.

Julie was interested. She realized that Ger was putting mindful communication into action when he interacted with coworkers and patients. She saw how mindfulness would make a difference in her communication with patients. With Ger as her guide, Julie learned to use mindful communication to build better bonds with her patients and address problems on the unit.

Consider This:

Do you purposely avoid speaking with certain patients, coworkers, or visitors on your ward? Do you shy away from conflict situations? Do you instantly take offence when someone speaks to you in a loud voice, or a demanding tone? Are you uncomfortable with silence? Have you ever laughed inappropriately at a comment a patient or coworker made, or a question they asked?

Mindful communication is about becoming aware of the ways you send information into the world. When you are conscious of the messages you project, you understand the effect that your words and actions have on others. Ger communicated in a way that helped people open up, avoiding conflict. Like him, you can replace mindlessness with mindfulness to open a channel for true connection to occur. When you create opportunities for reciprocal communication, you will feel a closer connection with others and respond compassionately.

With increased presence comes kindness and compassion—the nurse's calling cards. Your posture, tone of voice, and choice of words all communicate who you are and how you feel to the people you encounter every day. Even without words, you communicate through touch, body language, and facial expression.

How do you practice mindful communication? Thich Nhat Hanh described it perfectly: "Listen to your patient with only one purpose: to give him a chance to empty his heart and to suffer less. You may be the first person who has listened to him like this."[57]

Compassionate Communication in Nursing

Nursing is a synergistic profession. That is to say nurses should understand what their patients need by connecting with them, just as Ger did. This genuine connection reassures your patients that you care.

As an example of this synergy, let's look at Joe, a typical patient. When Joe arrives at your hospital, he is doubled over with pain and discomfort and is experiencing a heightened sense of helplessness. He feels terrified, anxious, confused, and embarrassed about what's going on in his body. He can't understand what's happening and is scared to surrender control to the doctors and nurses. If he experiences any coolness or misunderstanding from the staff, it will make him feel worse.

For the healing channels to open, you need to be able to understand where Joe is coming from—and not merely "go through the motions" with him. Medical treatment alone will not make Joe feel better—he also needs to feel understood. More than anything, your mindful presence will enable you to offer Joe what he needs.

Use your active listening skills to get in touch with what Joe is feeling. Help him feel heard by rephrasing his statements, mirroring his actions, and offering him encouraging prompts. If he says how scared he is, respond by acknowledging that it must be difficult to be so scared. By pausing and listening mindfully, you invite him to tell you more. As he talks, maintain eye contact, a friendly face, and open body posture.

As you listen, pay attention to your gut feelings. More than half the information in a conversation is typically communicated through body language. If you are distracted and not giving Joe your full attention, much of this potentially valuable information will be overlooked or missed entirely. In contrast, your mindful presence will help Joe to be more open and freely express himself.

You treat a disease, you win, you lose.
You treat a person, I guarantee you win—no matter the outcome.
—Patch Adams

Listening Mindfully

When did you last tap into the power of communication as a tool for healing and connection? Today's world is fast-paced and hyperconnected. You may feel compelled to say something at every moment. Society encourages us to tweet, blog, and network all the time, whether or not we have something to say. When you live in such an interactive world, it can be difficult to slow down and think before you speak.

Mindful listening has numerous benefits, including:

- *Focus.* How often have you missed the last thing someone said because your mind was elsewhere? At work, you might have difficulty focusing on your patient's concerns because you're preoccupied by your to-do list.

- *Information Gathering.* When patients feel heard, they are more likely to share vital information that may be important in understanding their symptoms. Also, when you are fully present, you are more likely to ask better questions. How many times have you gone back to a patient, shocked that they omitted an important detail of their illness, only to hear, "Well, you never asked"?

- *Seeing the Larger Picture.* Mindful listening helps you tune in to your patients in a way that makes you more likely to notice an unusual symptom or side effect.

The most basic and powerful way to connect to another person
is to listen. Just listen. Perhaps the most important thing
we ever give each other is our attention.

—Rachel Naomi Remen

When you next engage in conversation with a patient, colleague, or family member, practice mindful listening. In addition to becoming a better listener, this practice will help you to see the inner workings of your own mind more clearly.

Try This:
Mindful Listening

Practice mindful listening during a conversation. Make listening to this person the anchor for your attention in the same way you use your breath as an anchor in sitting meditation.

Don't assume you already know what the person is going to tell you. Instead, open a space within yourself where deep listening can take place.

Notice any tension in your body or mind and any impulse to jump in with unnecessary questions or commentary.

When judgments arise about what the person is saying, notice them and return to listening.

Listen for what is *not* being said—what the person is communicating nonverbally. When other thoughts or emotions pull at your attention, gently come back, and continue listening for the remainder of the conversation.

Notice whether the quality of the interaction feels different when you engage mindfully.

Journal Reflection:

After you try out this practice, reflect:

What did you notice in your own experience as you listened?

What did you notice about the other person?

Was it easy or difficult to listen in this way?

How was this different from the way you usually listen?

Earlier, you were introduced to mindful breathing and the body scan. You also learned how to practice being mindful of sounds and thoughts. Having reached this point in the book, you now have a good foundation for the formal sitting meditation that comes next.

Sitting meditation begins with mindful breathing, and then attention gradually expands to include the whole body, sounds, thoughts and emotions—finally expanding to a wide, open awareness. This is sometimes called *spacious awareness*, or *choiceless awareness* because you remain open and alert to whatever arises in your experience from moment to moment. This practice may seem more complex than any you have tried so far. You are learning to open up awareness and space and, ultimately, to rest in awareness itself. Try it out, remembering to cultivate patience as you go along. (You can access a guided audio recording of this practice by visiting www.nursingmindfully.com.)

Try This:
Open-Awareness Meditation

Settle into a comfortable posture for this sitting, with your back straight, chin tucked slightly under. Gradually bring your attention to your breathing, noticing the physical sensations in the lower abdomen as you breathe...noticing the rise and fall of the abdomen with each breath. Allow the breath to be your anchor, coming back to the breath when you notice your mind has wandered, bringing an attitude of kindness and patience to your experience.

Now gradually expand your awareness to include the sensations arising in your body as you breathe. Feel your whole body breathing.

From focusing on your breath and body, expand your attention now to include sounds—not forcing yourself to hear anything, just being open to the sounds around you, no matter how soft or loud...opening yourself up to the "soundscape," noticing loud and obvious sounds, as well as more subtle ones...noticing as well if there are moments when you don't hear anything.

Accept sounds as they are, as sensations, without striving to interpret them or identify where they are coming from. If you notice yourself thinking about what the sounds mean, gently bring your focus back to their sensory qualities: Is the sound loud? Soft? Is it deep? High-pitched? Notice sounds as they come and go from moment to moment.

Now gently let go of sounds, widening your awareness still further to include thoughts. Notice thoughts arising as images, sounds, memories...being aware of thoughts as they arise, as they linger, and dissolve...letting thoughts come and go as they will, just like clouds passing through a spacious sky. (cont'd)

When you find yourself involved in thoughts, gently step back and let them be, knowing they will pass. You can label the thought as "worrying," "planning," "problem-solving," or whatever it may be.

If a thought or an image arouses a strong emotion, pleasant or unpleasant, gently note what the emotion is, how intense it is—and then let it be. When you find it hard to do so, or your mind is too busy, gently return attention to your breath and body, letting this focus anchor your awareness.

When you feel ready, you can let let go of thoughts, sounds, and emotions, allowing the field of your awareness to open up to whatever arises from moment to moment. As you rest in open awareness, let your awareness be as wide, spacious and vast as the sky...simply noticing whatever arises in this expansive space. At times, you may notice sounds. At other times, there may be thoughts, emotions, or sensations. Any one may be predominant in your awareness for a time. Notice them arising and passing away, just like clouds passing through the sky. Sit and observe them as they drift into your awareness, lingering for a while and dissolving. Resting in the vastness of awareness itself. Witness the change in mind and body from moment to moment.

If you find your mind wandering, or busy, or you don't know where to place your attention, simply return to the breath at any time to stabilize your awareness.

When you feel ready to end the meditation, gently bring your attention back to the breath, feeling the rise and fall of the body as you breathe. As you end this session, acknowledge yourself for creating space in the busyness of your day for your own well-being, perhaps setting the intention to bring the spacious, open awareness you have cultivated into the rest of your day.

Question without Judgment

Every day, you work with patients. Some may be difficult and, although you may try hard to hide your irritation, they often sense your underlying attitude—even though you don't convey it directly through words.

When you are fully present—not lost in emotions or judgment—you ask questions and hear the answers more clearly. As a result, you win your patients' trust and cooperation, which translates into better care for them and an easier work environment for you.

This can be particularly important when a patient has an embarrassing problem they may not want to disclose—for example, erectile dysfunction can indicate other problems, such as heart disease, so it is important to know if your patient is affected. The only way to access such sensitive information is to be open and interested when asking about intimate details of your patient's health and lifestyle. Bear in mind, your patient is more likely to self-disclose when you are friendly and receptive.

You might find it challenging to be non-judging at times, especially if patients admit to behaviors you find offensive. If you withdraw, or display any type of disapproval in response to what they are confiding, they will often sense your judgment and shut down. You risk your patient withholding the very information you need to know to provide them the best care.

A nurse named Andrea discovered this the hard way. Andrea worked in a drug rehabilitation center and found it rewarding to help her patients move on with their lives. When they came to rehab, many patients were able to open up about what had brought them to this point in their lives. However, one patient was quite reticent, so Andrea decided to invest more time connecting with him one-on-one. During the course of their conversations, the man disclosed that he was a convicted child molester. Immediately, Andrea's body clenched and she became silent. "I messed up, man," the patient said. "I have so many regrets." At that point, Andrea couldn't think of anything to say and left the room. Later, once she got her anger under control, she tried to talk to the patient. However, by then the patient had completely withdrawn and would not talk to anyone. Even worse, he requested that Andrea be re-assigned away from him. Unfortunately, the patient's recovery took several steps backwards—he wouldn't take his meds, talk to his therapist, or participate in group therapy.

Mindful communication means letting go of judgment, which Andrea was unable to do initially. Yet no one is saying this is always easy.

Using "right speech" can be a challenge in general, but even more so in nursing. Why? Because when you work in stressful situations, dealing with people's fears and feelings of helplessness concerning their pain and illness, you may encounter volatile emotions and heightened reactions. Your patients and their families are distressed, worried, and anxious—and you present a convenient outlet for those fears. No doubt you have witnessed and experienced countless angry families act out toward staff, or patients who react in a rude, sarcastic manner despite the fact that you are trying to help them. Although challenging, it's at these difficult moments that being mindful of your reactions and your speech is most important.

Mindful communication is a powerful tool to help you respond skillfully in such situations. Communicating with awareness and kindness, and listening without judgment, are at the heart of good nursing practice and help you to establish a secure connection with your coworkers, your patients, and their families.

Practice Plan:

Practice mindful listening with your patients and coworkers this week, letting go of any tendency to judge.

Continue to cultivate goodwill for yourself and others through the practice of loving-kindness and compassion.

Keep up other aspects of your formal daily practice by mixing and alternating the practices of sitting, walking, and mindful movement in whatever ways you choose.

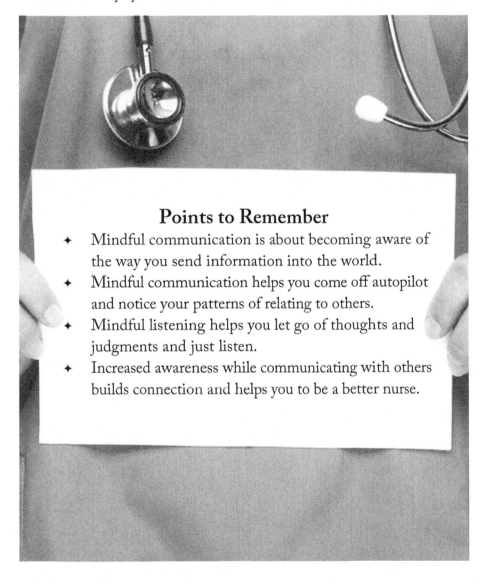

Points to Remember

+ Mindful communication is about becoming aware of the way you send information into the world.
+ Mindful communication helps you come off autopilot and notice your patterns of relating to others.
+ Mindful listening helps you let go of thoughts and judgments and just listen.
+ Increased awareness while communicating with others builds connection and helps you to be a better nurse.

CHAPTER EIGHTEEN

Working with Distractions, Preventing Errors

Over four hundred thousand preventable deaths occur each year as a result of medical errors. That's tantamount to killing the entire population of Miami, Florida, in one year—Sacramento, California, the next.

—Dr. Tom Muha

Emma worked in a busy pediatrics unit, one of the only facilities specializing in children for at least one hundred fifty miles. Her floor admitted the most critical children, which generated stress for Emma. Patient acuity was high and staffing low. Although this exacerbated the pressure for everyone, Emma smiled through the stress and kept going.

Emma was already caring for two critical patients when she heard that a critically injured toddler was on his way up to her floor. She was in a hurry to prepare the necessary supplies and medications for his admission, and she knew she needed to closely calculate the medications based on his anticipated weight. As she rushed, she kept looking out to see if the young trauma patient had arrived. Because she wasn't paying close attention to her calculation, she calculated a dose twice what the child should receive.

Emma did not realize she made a mistake until the child started to have difficulty breathing. She knew it was her fault and that it had happened because she was distracted. Had she focused on what she was doing, she would have gotten the right dose, and her patient would not have had to suffer because of her mistake.

Everybody makes mistakes. Most nurses know well that errors such as Emma's are all too common, but you might not know the actual statistics for medical errors. According to the National Research Council, in 2000 the US Institute of Medicine found that between forty-four thousand and ninety-eight thousand hospitalized patients die every year from medical errors.[58] Almost 17% of hospital admissions include at least one error, and over half of these are highly preventable.[59] Also, a report by the UK Department of Health found that 10% of patients admitted to hospitals in the United Kingdom suffer an adverse reaction, disability, or death due to an error made by medical staff.[60]

Consider This:

Have you ever made a medication error? Did you report it or hide it? Are you still living with the guilt? Have you ever forgotten to write down vital signs taken, and instead of redoing them, you just adlibbed numbers in your charting? Have you ever given a medication to a patient who was not wearing any ID but felt it was okay because you "recognized them" and you were in a hurry to finish the med pass?

Unfortunately, in the medical arena, errors—even seemingly minor ones—can have significant consequences. Mistakes can cause serious patient harm and even death.

Although errors can and do happen because we are human, we can strive to reduce them as much as possible. The primary causes of errors in nursing are distraction and stress. One Gallup poll estimated that 50% of a typical hospital's staff is "disengaged"—on autopilot—at work.[61] When autopilot thinking, stress, or some form of interruption takes your mind away from a task, you are more likely to make a mistake.

If you reduce your levels of distraction and stress, errors are less likely. Although a world without distractions and stressors is impossible, mindfulness can help by improving your attention and reducing your stress level—and as a result, you are less likely to make harmful mistakes.

When acting in a state of mindlessness, it is easy to be unaware of what both body and mind are doing (automatic pilot mode) and to operate dangerously in an already complex setting.

—*Is Mindful Reflective Practice the Way Forward to Reduce Medication Errors?* by Cinzia Pezzolesi, Maisoon Ghaleb, Andrzej Kostrzewski, and Soraya Dhillon

Hazards of Autopilot Mode

It is easy to slip into autopilot mode when you are distracted or have too much to do. On autopilot, you think less clearly as you move from task to task, underestimating the gravity of the problems you meet on your way. As a result, you may fail to respond to monitors, misinterpret vital signs, or pass the wrong meds.

To avoid drifting into autopilot, consider setting the ringer on your phone to regularly bring you back to the present. When the ringer reminds you, take a breath and connect with what you are doing in the moment.

It is particularly dangerous to be on autopilot when a patient is experiencing a changing medical condition. Pause and take a moment of mindful reflection before you act.

Try This:
Mindful Reflection

Mindful reflection can be accomplished by asking these few simple questions:

Am I actually doing what the patient needs?

Does this situation require intervention such as calling a doctor or calling a code?

Am I fully present for this patient right now or am I rushing through the procedure so I can move on to the next task?

Am I assuming I know what is wrong with the patient, or have I checked the evidence in front of me?

Journal Reflection:

Take a moment to reflect on any errors you have made in your nursing career.

To what do you attribute these errors?

What can you do, starting now, to prevent similar mistakes in the future?

Distraction wastes our energy. Concentration restores it.

—Sharon Salzberg

Avoiding Distractions during Medication Administration

Administering medications is the nursing activity most associated with errors. As it happens, it is also the most common activity in your daily routine.

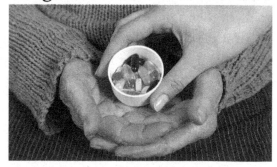

Jill Kremer, a cardiac nurse, made this observation: "The feeling of defeat often occurs in nursing, but it is never so acute as when you realize you made a mistake...and that mistake was a medication error. Even when the mistake is caught in time—but especially when it causes harm to the patient—it can rip apart a nurse's self-esteem. We are taught to do no harm, and most of the time we don't. We don't actively seek to harm. Yet we are not above mistakes. Nurses know their actions can have long-term repercussions for patients. That's why it's so tragic when we accidentally hurt someone."

Several issues can lead to medication administration errors: distractions by patients, family, and coworkers; autopilot mode; and overwhelming stress. One way to rise above this is to be mindful of the *five rights* when distributing meds.

Identifying the five rights is part of your training. Medication errors usually result from violation of one of these rights. No matter how many times you give a patient medication, keep the five rights in mind: right patient, right medication, right dosage, right route, and right time. Reciting them to yourself can be your mindfulness practice while you administer medications in any situation.

Try This:
Mindful Medication Administration

As you move between each patient, take a moment to center yourself.

Focus for a few seconds on your breath.

Become aware of the physical sensation of your feet on the floor.

Bring your mind back to the five rights.

When you reach each patient, ask yourself whether this is the right patient, the right medication, the right dosage, the right route, and the right time.

It only takes a second to reorient your thoughts, but that mere second of mindfulness can help you avoid serious medication errors.

At work each day, many things compete for your attention. This can be stressful, overwhelmingly at times. When you feel stressed, you might rush through the medication administration process and assume that some or even all of the five rights are correct without thoroughly checking.

In the end, if you don't pay full attention to what you are administering, you can and possibly will make a mistake. So when you get distracted, take a mindful breath and ease yourself into *being* mode to get back on track.

When you take a moment to move mindfully between patients, you break the cycle of stress and let go of any distressing thoughts or physical tension so you can be fully present—allowing yourself the time you need to make sure the five rights are indeed right.

Elements to Consider

Remembering the five rights helps to prevent mistakes. Make sure you verify the five rights as follows:

- *Patient identification.* With computer systems and barcodes, it is easy to scan an ID bracelet and accept the information it provides. But in some cases, ID bands are damaged, incorrect, or missing. To accurately identify a patient, you should verbally confirm identifiers such as a birth date and the name of the medication being administered. By doing this, you prevent mistakes as you build your relationship with each patient.

- *Drug information.* Attend to the next four rights by making certain you are giving the right medication, in the right dosage, in the right route, at the right time.

Since it is easy to confuse drugs, particularly when the names or labels are similar, always take a moment to check the label. Mislabeled medications can cause grave errors. Before administering any drug, make sure the label is correct and that you are giving the patient the correct medication, concentration, dose, and route. Take that extra second to be mindful and avoid accidentally administering the wrong meds.

Pay particular attention to the technology used to deliver medications. Multi-channel and patient-controlled pumps are frequently used and offer even more opportunities for errors. It's important to always follow the same process when connecting or disconnecting fluids and medications to avoid fluid, air, or medication boluses. Paying careful attention to the task will prevent errors and minimize danger to patients.

Nurses are expected to stay organized, but if your unit is in perpetual chaos, that's not an easy thing to do. It can be difficult to give medications properly in small, messy, poorly lit rooms. Do what you can to clean and organize the front desk, work areas, and the patient rooms on your floor. Organized workspaces help prevent errors.

You can also prevent medication errors by educating patients. Talk to them about their medication as you administer it. If they know which medications they are taking, what they are for, and what they look like, they can do their part to prevent errors. Always tell your patients what you are giving them when you hand them the medicine cup or hang a piggyback. When your patient knows what's going on, they can provide the last check, helping you avoid errors.

Overcome Distractions

Whenever you dispense medications, make sure your environment is as free of distractions as possible—although this can prove challenging in hectic or chaotic facilities.

Patients can be one of your biggest distractions during medication administration. While you may be trying to focus mindfully on the five rights, your patient may be interested in chatting with you about an issue troubling them, such as chest pain, or a coughing fit. Of course, this makes it difficult to focus on their meds.

Try This:
Mindful Interaction

As you greet your patient during medication rounds, take a moment to give them your undivided attention. Listen, and reassure them that you will act on their concerns.

Then ask them to give you a few moments to concentrate so that you can administer their meds correctly. When you are finished, you can resume talking.

Sometimes other patients will distract you during medication administration. If another patient or family member experiences a medical emergency, stop what you are doing and attend to the emergency, but afterwards, bring your attention back to your first patient. Start your interaction again from the beginning, taking time to work mindfully through the protocols.

No matter what you are doing, it is easy to become momentarily distracted. Your fellow nurses, nurses' aides, and doctors can distract you, and regrettably, even momentary inattention can potentially lead to a serious mistake.

Take the case of Luke Carlson who worked in an orthopedic ward. Standing at the narcotics dispenser, Luke counted the pills left in the drawer. While he was counting, a CNA called his name, saying a doctor was on the phone for him. Not wanting to keep the doctor waiting, he shoved the narcs back in the drawer and quickly went to take the call.

It wasn't until he was about to give a patient his pain medicine that the error came up in the system. The count was off—the patient's pain pill had ended up in Luke's pocket! Luke's stomach tightened. Sweat beaded on his forehead. With shaking hands, he dialed the pharmacy and explained what happened. They came and reset the machine. Luke realized that if he hadn't been interrupted, the med-count error would not have occurred.

Luke's experience is not unique. Nurses face frequent interruptions. In fact, on average, nurses are interrupted and distracted as frequently as once every two minutes while administering medication.[62] That is an incredible litany of distractions when you think about it! If that weren't bad enough, there is a significant (12.7%) increase in the risk of a medication error with each interruption, and when a nurse is interrupted six times, the error rate triples.[63]

One way to avoid distractions by coworkers and other personnel is to post signs near medication preparation areas warning others not to distract you while you are preparing or administering meds. You can also politely tell coworkers you are currently busy and will get back to them when the job is complete. Some interruptions are unavoidable, such as medical emergencies and urgent phone calls, but at least you *can* stem routine interruptions until after you've prepared your patients' medication.

The next time you are distracted by colleagues or patients while administering medications, try the STOP practice before proceeding with your task.

S.T.O.P.

Stop
Take a breath
Observe
Proceed

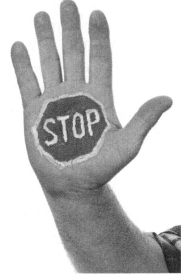

Try This:
STOP Practice

S top what you are doing.

T ake a breath, following your breath as it comes in and out of your nose.

O bserve your physical sensations, thoughts, and emotions. Are you aware of any tension? Take some mindful breaths.

P roceed once you feel calmer and more centered. Replay the five rights in your mind, giving each one considered attention before moving on to the next.

It may seem like an impossible feat to use the STOP practice every time you encounter an interruption, but with practice, you will find yourself able to stop, reorient yourself in a matter of seconds, and replay those five rights in your head.

Charting

When charting, you will meet many of the same distractions that you encounter during med pass. How many distractions you face will depend on where you chart, how you chart, and who is around you during that time. Of course, it will also vary with your work environment.

Clinical environments—such as the operating room, pediatric ward, medical-surgical units, and the emergency room—tend to be at high-risk for errors caused by distraction and interruptions. On average, emergency room nurses are interrupted more than ten times an hour.[64]

Not only that—fully 90% of interruption-related errors that medical and surgical nurses experienced have been traced to loss of focus and concentration, and resulted in delays in treatment.[65] These errors often happened during patient care procedures, medication administration, or documentation.

This was something that Nurse Joan Gardner discovered for herself while working with patients on a stroke unit. Charting was a job that Joan usually saved for the end of her shift. Although it was difficult to carve out time to do something as stationary as charting, Joan knew that when details aren't charted immediately, it's easy to forget them by the end of the shift.

One day, Joan's patient had high blood pressure. Although she called the doctor and got the situation under control, she didn't remember to record it when she charted at the end of her shift. Her notes didn't reflect the hypertensive event, and the patient's blood pressure spiked again after Joan went home.

When the relief nurse pulled up Joan's notes, she found no mention of high blood pressure, although the vitals entered by the CNAs clearly showed it had spiked earlier during her shift. The relief nurse did her best to make sense of Joan's notes. Eventually, she discovered that the patient had high blood pressure earlier and that although Joan had taken care of the situation, she had neglected to chart it.

In the end, Joan was called into the manager's office and had to make a late entry into the computer, documenting how she took care of the crisis. Although she wasn't punished, her manager was stern. But her manager's reaction didn't feel half as bad to Joan as did the knowledge that, due to her distraction, she hadn't fulfilled her duty to the patient.

Charting errors such as Joan's can lead to a patient experiencing a crisis. If you neglect to chart a change in vital signs because you were distracted, your patient could suffer. You will not only have to contend with the crisis but also cope with the emotional trauma from having made the error. For certain, no one wants that.

Whether charting in or near a patient's room or at the nurses' station, you will inevitably be exposed to many distractions: your patient may want to chat with you, family members may want to ask questions, or your fellow health professionals and visitors may take the opportunity to chat or ask for directions because they mistakenly think you're available to socialize.

Instead, find a quiet place on your unit and give full attention to the task, taking a moment to center yourself before you begin. If you have to stop midway, take a few mindful breaths on your return and resume the task.

Remember that it only takes a minute to stop and ground yourself.

Stress as a Distraction

Another common distraction is overwhelming stress. Often you may want to postpone charting or get it over and done with as quickly as possible because there are so many other demands on your time. As a result, charting may be left until the shift end, a time more convenient for the patient but decidedly less convenient for the nurse. If a lot has happened, you can be charting long after your shift is over. Tired, stressed, and anxious to get home, you may rush the process— and the stress of rushing can cause you to make errors and omissions.

If you leave charting until shift end, like Joan did, you may not be able to recall everything that happened. No matter how fastidious you were about taking notes, you might be unable to remember certain details of what happened twelve, ten, or even six hours before, and to recall exactly what you were thinking or how the patient looked. For this reason, it is helpful to chart mindfully as you go, rather than saving it for the end of your day. This will help you to reduce errors.

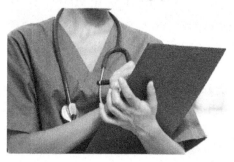

Handling Distractions during Emergencies

Distractions are a particularly critical problem during emergencies, as the environment is one that is always subject to change in a split second. It is easy, for example, for a patient's heart monitor to distract you when it changes from one rhythm to another, when it gives false information, or when you fixate on the rhythm and not the causes behind it. If something knocks you off-course, you may have a hard time getting back to the ACLS (advanced cardiac life support) algorithms. Chaos can add to the difficulty, increasing your stress levels as well as the likelihood the patient will suffer.

Some medical professionals don't handle the frantic pace and demands of emergencies as well as others, and these coworkers can easily distract you and pull you off balance. Nevertheless, you can regain your composure by taking a mindful breath before tackling an emergency. Focus on the ACLS algorithms and your role. In a code, all team members have their own responsibilities. If you focus on your assigned job—and avoid multitasking—it is easier to pay attention to what *needs* your attention.

At times the source of your distraction may be your patients. They may be afraid, or their condition may rapidly change, causing you to change treatment directions. If you find yourself jumping steps in the protocols, mentally pause and take a moment to breathe. Then, start over, working your way through the appropriate algorithm or policy.

Nurses are called upon to think critically and react quickly to whatever the situation, and this requires that you remain mindful during the crisis at hand. For example, when a patient presents with crushing chest pain, you need to administer oxygen, nitroglycerin, aspirin, and morphine and also take and evaluate the EKG. As the patient improves or deteriorates going through the chest pain, dysrhythmia, and cardiac arrest phases, you need to stay focused on the nursing process: assess, diagnose, plan, implement, evaluate, and repeat.[66]

Refocusing based on a patient's rapidly changing presentation is often difficult, even confusing, and this is when mistakes can occur. As you grapple with the constant changes, working as swiftly as you can, perhaps you don't notice critical changes in patient acuity or changes in the EKG or don't see the unexpected reaction to the medication administered.

In an emergency, a cascade of bodily processes kicks in quickly: your breathing becomes rapid and shallow, and your heart rate increases while your mind races to determine the best course of action. In the end, you struggle to concentrate, or respond with purpose, to the patient's rapidly changing status. Whenever you have a stress reaction like this, you become less efficient.

When you find yourself in panic mode, mindfulness can help in two ways: reducing your stress symptoms and allowing clarity of thought, but to access these benefits, you need to pause briefly.

The pause may last only a second or two. If you use those seconds well, that mental reset can have a powerful impact on what happens next. It will help you become grounded, so you can respond, rather than react, to the situation.

Here is a practice that takes only a few seconds to do, yet helps you center yourself when panic threatens:

Try This:
Two Feet, One Breath

Focus your attention on the sensations in your feet as they make contact with the floor. This helps to slow down your thought process and ground your mind.

Take one deep breath, breathe slowly, in and out through your nose.

As your mind becomes calmer and more focused, proceed with the protocol.

If you do this practice routinely in less stressful circumstances, in time, you will be able to draw on it in chaotic situations, when you need it most. Then you can re-ground yourself in a matter of seconds.

There is no way to avoid the inevitable distractions, stress, and mistakes that are a part of every nurse's life. When you lose your concentration or get caught in pressured circumstances, the resulting confusion, however momentary, means that you are more apt to slip up, and every mistake can feel like a personal failure. Mindfulness is the antidote to this problem.

The more you practice in your everyday life, the easier it will be for you to be centered during medical emergencies and other challenging situations. In time, you will have more internal stability and be able to switch effortlessly to a mindful mode when you need it most, and proceed in a calm and organized fashion.

Although mindful practice cannot prevent all errors, it can reduce the amount of time you spend in autopilot mode, make you more aware of your surroundings, and improve your attention so that your patients receive the best possible care.

Practice Plan:

Pay particular attention this week to working mindfully with distractions and interruptions in your working environment. Use the STOP practice following interruptions. Continue to devote at least thirty minutes daily to your formal practice, combining and/or mixing practices as you choose. Reflect on your experience of your formal practice so far.

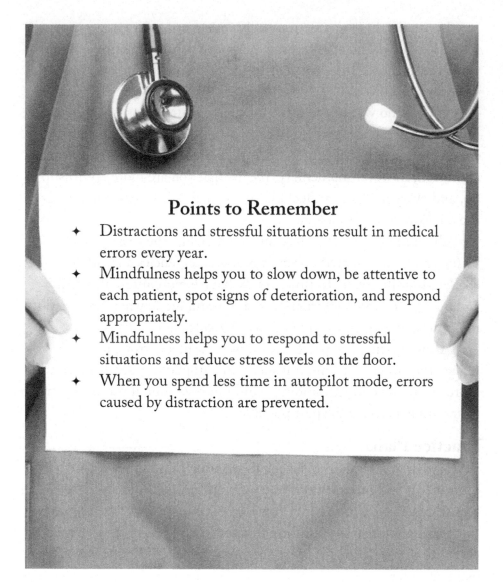

Points to Remember

+ Distractions and stressful situations result in medical errors every year.
+ Mindfulness helps you to slow down, be attentive to each patient, spot signs of deterioration, and respond appropriately.
+ Mindfulness helps you to respond to stressful situations and reduce stress levels on the floor.
+ When you spend less time in autopilot mode, errors caused by distraction are prevented.

CHAPTER NINETEEN

The Mindful Handover Report

When information is missed in patient handovers, people die.
—Mary Jane Wilson

By the end of a long shift, most nurses want nothing more than to go somewhere to sit down, relax, and rest their busy minds and tired bodies. Before that much-needed respite, however, there is one last hurdle between them and imminent freedom: the handover or handover report.

For some nurses, this last task is merely an afterthought after completing a long list of duties. A closer look at hospital incident reports, however, shows that around 80% of serious medical errors happen due to miscommunications during handover reports.[67]

Take the case of Deirdre Gilbert, a first-year RN who had been working the floor for several months. The nurse before her, rushing to punch out and avoid overtime, raced through his handover report. He told Deirdre that Mrs. R in Bed 10 was experiencing pain in her calf and that he had given her the prescribed pain medicine. However, in his haste, he failed to mention that Mrs. R's calf was red and slightly swollen, or that she was on Coumadin.

As Deirdre's shift progressed, Mrs. R's leg continued to swell and redden. She could barely move her foot. Within an hour, she was experiencing shortness of breath. Deirdre called the doctor, who ordered an ultrasound. It revealed a deep-vein thrombosis in the leg. A subsequent CT scan showed that Mrs. R now had a clot in her lungs.

If the previous RN had known the patient's background and communicated it to Deirdre, this problem could have been resolved before it evolved into a life-threatening pulmonary embolism. As this case study shows, clinical handovers are high-risk situations for patient safety. In this instance, the failure to fully communicate the patient's symptoms and history led to a poor outcome for the patient.

Errors due to ineffective handovers have led to delays in diagnosis and treatment, unnecessary tests and treatments, incorrect patient treatment, increases in the length of hospital stay, patient complaints, and malpractice claims. Had all parties involved communicated effectively, most of these errors could easily have been prevented.[68]

Consider This:

Have you ever been so tired at the end of a shift that you purposefully left information out of your report, feeling that the nurse coming on duty would likely figure it out? Has a patient of yours ever suffered an adverse reaction or new health problem because, in your haste to depart work, you neglected to pass on certain information or observations? Have you ever had to deal with a crisis situation because a coworker forgot to properly report a patient's condition to you?

As the frontline in care delivery, you bear a crucial responsibility to ensure your patients receive consistent quality care. Undoubtedly the handover report plays an essential role in this, benefitting the patients entrusted to your care, who, in turn, you entrust to your colleagues. A properly conducted handover report actually protects you, too. Most of all, the handover ties up loose ends and makes sure critical work is delegated to the right people so it gets done correctly and on time.

For the nurse going off duty, the handover is a chance to clean off your "desk" for the day. How many times have you left your workplace only to be bothered by a nagging feeling that you left something undone? In a field where mistakes can compromise comfort and safety, a good handover report provides you with a welcome sense of closure, and, once you achieve that closure, you can make the most of your time off.

On the other hand, when you are the nurse on the receiving end of the handover, having the necessary critical information makes the shift easier to handle, saving you from costly mistakes and false starts.

To allow time and space for handover is crucial so that nurses have a place to debrief and reflect on the nursing shift. This creates a professional space to give away their workload free from outsider comment.

—Sharyn Wallis

Mindful Communication

Although the handover report is crucial to ensuring patient safety and continuity of care, it is surprising that most training programs neglect to focus on or develop this skill. The Joint Commission International, widely considered the gold standard for global healthcare accreditation, only recently considered handover communication a focal area for patient safety.[69] Even when institutional policy does not recognize the importance of handover communication, being mindful during this time is a worthwhile and rewarding habit to cultivate.

Also referred to as patient-care transfer, the College of Nurses of Ontario defined the handover as "an interactive process of transferring patient-specific information from one caregiver to another or from one team to another for the purpose of ensuring the continuity and safety of the patient's care."[70] The main purpose of the handover report is to transfer all the information the receiving nurse or team needs to effectively take over a patient's care. Yet, giving—and receiving—a handover report requires more than a mere mechanical transfer of information.

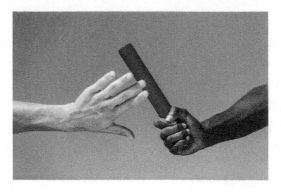

The keyword for handovers is *interactive*, and the goal should not be to rattle off a list of things that should or should not be done during the next shift. Rather, a handover should be a collaborative task. This is where mindfulness comes in. When you are mindful, you think critically and look at the big picture. This means having a clear understanding of your role as a member of your patient's medical team. More than any other care provider on the team, you are involved with many dimensions of your patient's care—not just the medical aspects, but also the emotional and physical dimensions. On an interactive level, your contribution can be great.

Denise Douglas loved her position as a nurse in the post-anesthesia care unit. When coming on shift, she reviewed all the orders and the latest blood work for her patients. To get a full report, Denise would ask the outgoing shift nurse astute questions about how the patient's vitals had been, if the patient still needed oxygen or was on room air, or if the surgical site showed any signs of infection. Some of Denise's coworkers were instead very cavalier about giving the patient report, but Denise always insisted on reviewing the condition and needs of patients from head-to-toe—both when coming on shift and when leaving. As a result, many of the more experienced nurses in the unit appreciated Denise's thorough approach to report, and the newer nurses learned a lot from her attention to detail.

Whether you are delivering or receiving a handover report, mindful communication ensures the handover is effective. Before the handover, take some time to stand back from the immediate details of your patient's care and see the bigger picture.

Try This:
Handover Reflection
Ask yourself the following questions at the time of handover:

Who is the patient?

What is their condition and medical history?

What does my colleague need to know (or what do I need to know) in order to deliver the best possible care?

Guidelines for Giving a Handover

When you conduct the handover, pay attention to the following to make sure the handover is efficient:

Communicate—don't just recite. As the person delivering the handover report, you'll do most of the talking. This means you set the tone of the handover interaction. Rather than simply staring at the receiving nurse while you tonelessly and impatiently prattle off a list of facts and numbers, make it a real conversation. When you interact in a mindful way, your coworkers will be encouraged to engage more and ask questions, if needed.

Be aware of nonverbal cues that indicate how the other person is processing what you are saying. For instance, if the other person is furiously writing down the information, then talk a little more slowly to let them catch up. On the other hand, if the receiving nurse seems to have missed the significance of something you think is important, then emphasize it by repeating it. Be sure to verify that this person understands all the important information.

Know what you have to say beforehand. Just as you would never call a doctor for a consult without first having all the pertinent data in front of you, always ensure you fully prepare for the handover. Remember that your handover report is designed to tie up all the loose ends from your shift, so make sure it covers all the bases. This is especially important when it comes to changes in the patient's condition, adjustments in medication orders, and preparations for medical procedures. To help you remember every focus area you need to include in the report, use a mental checklist or keep a written one handy. Again, use the same checklist every time, so you will be much less likely to leave out anything significant.

Deliver the most important information at the beginning. By giving the most important information at the start, you help your colleagues to prioritize the patient's needs. Usually, this information includes the patient's chief complaint, symptoms, lab results that need monitoring, and changes in medication. Important information might also include critical interventions and preps that must be done, as well as anything else you feel is relevant.

Welcome the opportunity to provide clarification or answers. After delivering your handover, ask whether your colleague needs to know anything else. This gives the receiving nurse a welcome chance to ask you to repeat something or give information you might have missed. Inviting feedback in an approachable, receptive way makes it clear that you are open to questions or requests for further information.

You would be surprised by how often receiving nurses hold back from asking questions because they know the outgoing nurse is anxious to leave. This is especially true when the outgoing nurse is the more senior of the two.

Focus on continuity. Although shifts may be neatly divided into a certain number of hours, patient events and nursing tasks are not organized in the same way. In fact, you'll often find things that began on a previous shift roll over to the next shift. Delivering safe and effective patient care is a team effort. Be aware of tasks and events that happened before your shift, as well as those that will (or should) happen after you leave, and remember to integrate this information into your handover report.

Receiving the handover report is your first task as soon as you get to work, and it sets the tone for the rest of your shift. An end-of-shift handover is where you dot all your i's and cross all your t's, and it lets you leave work with the peace of mind that your patients are being well cared for. Although the handover is a shift change routine, you need to be mentally on your toes during it—both at the beginning of your shift and at the end—as much vital information is communicated within a short timeframe.

Journal Reflection:

Take a few moments to reflect on how fully you engage during handovers. How present do you normally feel during the handover? Do you often find yourself leaning into the next moment, with your thoughts elsewhere? Or does your experience vary widely from day to day?

Considerations When Receiving a Handover

As the receiving nurse during a handover, you want the true clinical picture for every patient that will be in your care. So pay attention to the following:

Focus. Handovers can be overwhelming and stressful when you only have a few minutes and other work is calling for your attention. The more hectic a shift, the more crucial a thorough handover report becomes. Before you dive into the endless fray of tasks that await you, make sure you know everything necessary to make the right judgment calls during your shift. Remember to see every minute you engage with the handover report as time well spent; pay attention and listen mindfully. Focus on the person delivering the handover and put other things out of your mind for the moment. Whenever you notice your attention has been hijacked by things to do, take a slow, deep breath, renew eye contact with the other care provider, and bring yourself right back to the here and now.

Speak up. The handover is a dynamic process of communication between you and the outgoing medical care provider. It is up to you to ensure that you have all the information you need. Don't hesitate to ask questions or voice your concerns, even if you are less experienced or less senior than the person giving the report. Take a mindful breath and connect with the questions you need to ask to ensure a safe handover.

Use open-ended anticipatory questions, such as: What are you concerned about? What could go wrong here? Speaking out is part of advocating for your patients' safety and comfort.

Have ready a checklist of what you need to know. With so much information to cover during the handover, it is easy to overlook something important. However, your mindful presence will help you to avoid overlooking vital information. Take a moment in advance of the handover to get in touch with the information you need, and develop a checklist to ensure the report covers everything.

This checklist does not have to be complex or sophisticated; a simple mnemonic tool may suffice. For example, the mnemonic PMEDS will help you account for precautions, medications, exams, diet, and signs/symptoms; or you can devise your own quick checklist. Keep it handy by printing it out on a small card that you can carry in your pocket.

Prioritize drug information. Familiarity with your patient's medications, their contraindications, interactions, and side effects will provide you with insight into the patients' clinical condition and acuity.

Arrange for bedside handover reports when possible. While not always possible in certain settings, bedside handovers can help prevent confusion and misinformation. They also save you time because you can conduct an initial shift assessment at the same time. Likewise, the patient or any family members present can promptly clarify any inconsistent information given in the report. You can also conveniently conduct patient safety checks, like confirming identification and allergy bands and IV fluids. Another advantage of the bedside handover report is that it lets you connect with your patient. That way, you feel more involved in their care from the onset of your shift.

Bedside shift reports have been found to increase patient involvement and satisfaction, boost nursing teamwork and accountability, and improve the effectiveness of communication among caregivers.
— *Nurse Shift Report,* by Cherri D. Anderson
and Ruthie R. Mangino

Without doubt, the handover report is one of the most underappreciated tools for patient safety. Although typically viewed as a routine task—one that might appear redundant with the use of so many electronic methods of communication (care plans, charting, ordering, and results reporting)—the handover report has a function that other reports cannot deliver—it facilitates intelligent interaction between two medical care providers.

Whether you deliver or receive the handover report, mindful communication during handovers is essential and can significantly reduce the risk of errors and accidents during your shift and the ones that follow.

Practice Plan:

Make it part of your regular practice to do the three-step breathing space before you engage in the handover, and observe the quality of your attention during the handover. Continue your formal practice this week, mixing the various practices you have learned in any way you choose. Reflect on how your formal practice is going. What obstacles and challenges are you encountering, and how can you work with them?

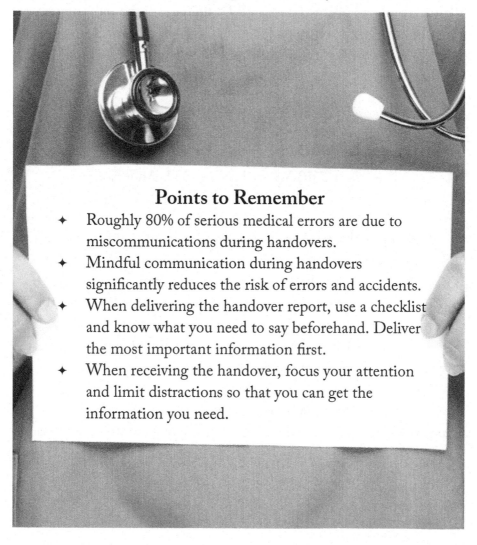

Points to Remember

+ Roughly 80% of serious medical errors are due to miscommunications during handovers.
+ Mindful communication during handovers significantly reduces the risk of errors and accidents.
+ When delivering the handover report, use a checklist and know what you need to say beforehand. Deliver the most important information first.
+ When receiving the handover, focus your attention and limit distractions so that you can get the information you need.

CHAPTER TWENTY

The Challenge
of Advancing Technology

With awareness and mindfulness, technology can be a friend, not a foe.
—Kenley Neufeld

Martha Nichols had been a nurse for thirty years. Over those three decades, she had seen changes on the med-surg unit where she worked. Since her fulfillment in nursing came from interacting with her patients, she had no aspirations to move to a different unit or to pursue further education.

Of course, nursing had changed quite a lot since Martha started. The demands of technology kept creeping into her nursing role, and using it left her less time to connect with her patients. Now, she did all her charting on the computer, checking off boxes on the screen. When she started her nursing career, charting was done by hand. To give medications now, she had to scan them into the computer and then scan the patient's bracelet. Although this system helped to reduce errors and ensure the five rights were met, she often found herself more engaged with the computer than with her patient.

Martha considered herself an intelligent, well-trained nurse. Although she had never been formally taught how to use the computer interface, she learned by trial and error. She also made countless calls to the technical service for assistance.

As the demands of technology increased, Martha became disillusioned with this aspect of her work. Instead of focusing on patient care, she spent more time on the computer, and she wasn't always certain she was even getting it right. In the end, Martha grew to hate technology—she felt it added to the stress of her shift and stole valuable time from her patients. She missed how she practiced nursing initially, when she had time to connect with her patients, free from the strain of technology.

The problem wasn't that Martha was too set in her ways to change, but that she felt stressed trying to keep up with the ever-changing demands of new technology in the absence of adequate support. On the verge of burnout, Martha felt that if something didn't change soon, she would have to take early retirement.

Martha's situation was not exceptional. The reality is that the nursing profession is immersed in new technology. Patients are hooked up to a plethora of electronic machines: automatic IV-pumps, telemetry heart monitoring, and vital-sign machines. If you work in critical care, you must process information from numerous complex gadgets attached to your patients. In addition, medications are now often delivered by scanning computer systems, and many facilities require nurses to carry cell phones to stay in touch with patients and doctors.

Although technology is unquestionably helpful and makes nursing easier in some respects than it was twenty years ago, attention to the patient can sometimes get lost. When devices compete for your focus, it can be harder, not easier, to do your job well.

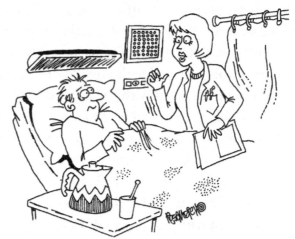

"We ran your symptoms through the computer and it caused a virus that shut down the internet!"

Consider This:

Have you avoided charting certain entries because you are slow at inputting to a computer? Have you missed inputting vital information about a patient because it was not on the check list used to collect data, and now you feel it is too late, or too time consuming, to go back and make late entries? Have you ever ignored a patient complaint because the monitor indicated they were fine?

The solution is to become mindful when you're using technology. How? Start by setting the intention to prioritize interaction with your patient over machines, using technology as the adjunct it was designed to be.

In Plum Village, France, the home of Vietnamese monk Thich Nhat Hanh, a mindfulness bell rings at random intervals during the day. The monks stop what they are doing and take a mindful breath when they hear the bell. The bell is their wakeup call to come back to being in the moment.

In the midst of your workday, you can use every experience you have with technology—whether a ringing phone, a beeping monitor, or a screen—as your mindfulness bell. When you hear these sounds, pay attention and respond appropriately. Notice the reactions in your body (clenching in the belly, tension in the temples) and any sense of wanting to push the sound away or resist it. Allow the reactivity to fall away on the out breath, and come back to the here and now.

Meditation is the ultimate mobile device; you can use it anywhere, anytime, unobtrusively.

—Sharon Salzberg

Patient-Centered Charting

All interactions with patients now include electronic interface. In theory, the use of technology frees up time that can be spent attending to your patient. In reality, though, technology can inadvertently become a barrier between nurse and patient, making it difficult to initiate and maintain the connection necessary for a patient's well-being and care.

For instance, most admission paperwork is now a checklist that you can breeze through once you know it well enough. Does your patient have diabetes? Check yes or no. Is he or she in pain? If so, what is the rating? How much thought do you give their responses when you're typing them in? For instance, are you absorbing the fact that your patient has an 8 out of 10 pain score or just absently noting it in your haste to move onto the next task?

When you don't give proper attention to all the facts a patient presents, you can miss something crucial. If your patient's pain score is 8 out of 10, then you need to find out why. Merely plugging in the information will not ensure the patient receives appropriate care.

It can be difficult to stay focused on the patient while you enter mountains of data into the computer system. Worse, if you focus on the screen rather on than the patient, he or she feels left out of the loop.

To combat this, consciously shift your focus away from the monitor, redirect your attention back to the patient, and observe their condition. Noticing something as simple as skin color can indicate how a patient is feeling. For example, a paler than normal complexion might suggest that your patient is in pain, while a patient with blue lips might be having trouble breathing. If you rush through your interaction, you could miss this vital information.

Although you may sigh and think you don't have time to pay attention in this way, in truth, it is easier than you think. For one thing, it only takes a few seconds to ask a question. Patients can be intuitive, and if you give them the impression that you are too busy or stressed to listen properly, they may not answer your questions truthfully or fully.

If they sense you're distracted, dismissive, or anxious to move on, they might be reluctant to open up and disclose pertinent information.

Try This:
Mindful Encounter

As you prepare to type up a patient's information, take a moment to gather yourself.

Put down the scanner, the tablet, the mouse, or the phone.

Look at the patient as if they were a family member and ask how they are doing.

Involve the Patient in Their Care through Technology

Old-school nurses like Martha, whom you read about earlier, may find the use of technology intrusive, preferring to talk to patients instead of using the tools at hand, while new-school nurses may rely too heavily and readily on technology.

You can integrate these two approaches to make patient care most efficient. To do this, engage your patient with the technology, using it as a teaching tool by turning the monitor toward them so they can see their chart. If the cholesterol is high, point out the numbers and let the patient see the normal range, explaining everything in simple terms. Seeing hard evidence on the computer screen can influence your patient and engage them more actively in their own healing process.

The benefits of technology in patient care unquestionably far outweigh its shortcomings. Provided you take time to focus on the patient, technology can be a powerful tool. A range of machines provides information to all professionals who come

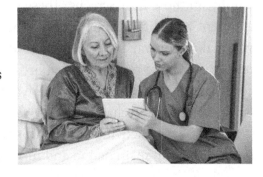

in contact with the patient, crystallizing patient goals and helping to reduce errors. The key is to use technology to help the patient, never forgetting that you are there *to connect with the person*, not the machine.

Try This:
Mindful Use of Computers

You head to a patient's room to check on their beeping IV pump. As you approach their room, you ground yourself by feeling your feet in contact with the floor and taking a slow, deep breath.

You pause and knock before entering, feeling your knuckles as they tap on the door. In these first moments, your focus is on the patient and not on technology.

Once you establish rapport, inform the patient that you will be using the computer to make notes on their care.

If you have a portable computer, tilt the screen in their direction when you record your observations.

Treat the Patient, Not the Monitor

A popular axiom, the saying "treat the patient, not the monitor" has become increasingly difficult to accomplish in modern nursing due to the countless pieces of electronics, machines, and technology used in healthcare facilities.

If you work on a floor with monitors such as telemetry, ICU, and step-down, for example, then you know how easy it is to focus wholly on those little screens. These days, you can often check on a patient's condition from the doorway by scanning the monitor as you make your way to the next task. With telemetry, you don't even need to go into a patient's room, because their rhythms are sent via computer directly to the desk where a monitor tech or another nurse is watching for any changes.

However, practicing nursing this way presents a serious problem as monitors can malfunction and furnish false information. Minute changes in rate and rhythm may not be clear on the monitor or may not be seen until the patient is physically symptomatic. Consequently, to put a monitor's results in proper context, it's important to take time to look directly at the patient in the bed.

Gavin Woods, a nurse who worked in a telemetry unit, told me how he learned to never rely solely on monitor readings. Gavin took pride in being able to read the rhythms that transmitted to the nurse's station. The computer would alert him whenever a patient's rhythm changed, freeing him to continue charting. One morning, he heard loud snoring sounds coming from a patient's room, but, when he checked the monitor, the patient's rhythm seemed fine, only a little slower.

Gavin was momentarily reassured but after a couple of minutes, he felt uneasy and strode down the hall, following the sound. To his shock, he found the patient with blue lips and breathing irregular, snoring gasps. Immediately, Gavin ran into the room and started CPR, calling for help from the other nurses.

Despite the normal rhythms showing on the monitor, the patient's heart rate was decreasing which, without intervention, would have resulted in death. If Gavin had relied solely on the monitor and not checked the patient in person, there might have been a tragic outcome.

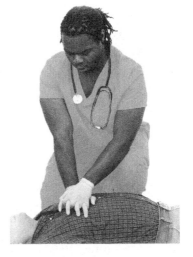

When you're busy, do you rely on the monitor as a substitute rather than using it as the complementary tool it's meant to be? Like Gavin, you need to check not just the monitor, but also the patient in person. Likewise, before you check the monitor, check in with yourself, noticing if your attention is focused or scattered.

Alarm Fatigue

The beeping heart monitor goes off yet again and you automatically silence it. Then it starts up a few seconds later and you silence it again, this time stabbing your finger against the button. It beeps a third time. Exasperated, you look at the monitor. It is not an error. Your patient is tachycardic.

There are so many alarms going off throughout the unit at any given moment: call bells, IV pump alarms, vital sign machines, heart monitors, pulse oximeters, and more. As a result, it's easy to mindlessly press the silence button since the cacophony can be too much at times. Who could blame you for wanting to silence all that noise?

Unfortunately, this is a dangerous practice, and it has a name: alarm fatigue. When you press the silence button, you assume you know exactly what is going on or not going on with a patient. But do you?

You might walk into a patient's room, silence a monitor, and walk out without a word. Sometimes you silence alarms from the desk, but what about your patient? If you enter a room because something is ringing, pause and talk to the patient while you are there. Maybe they need something. Maybe they need *you*. Take a moment to look at the screen. What is it saying? Do you need to investigate the ringing further? Look at the patient and see whether the monitor reading matches their condition.

Above all, do this *before* you silence the alarm. If you don't, your patient could suffer.

Try This:
Mindfulness Bell

Relate to the technology in your workplace as mindfulness bells, using certain sounds as wakeup calls. Whenever an electronic device alerts you to a potential problem, pause and take a breath, bringing awareness to the sound, and respond mindfully.

Journal Reflection:

How do you relate to technology in your workplace?

In what way does using it affect your mental and emotional state, as well as your body sensations?

Consider how the practices described in this chapter can help you to be mindful when using technology at work.

For better or worse, technology is here to stay. What's more, it can benefit you by streamlining your workflow, preventing errors, and helping you to keep a close eye on a patient's condition. However, it can also create a barrier to connection, which is unfortunate given that the relationship with your patients is paramount in nursing.

The answer is not for us to get rid of technology but to learn how to work with it mindfully. By using technology as a tool while taking every opportunity to be present with your patients, you ensure that technology enhances rather than detracts from your nursing practice. Clearly, when you use technology mindfully, you can provide the best care possible.

Practice Plan:

This week, notice your thoughts, feelings, and body sensations as you interact with technology at work. Be aware of your reactions, and in moments of frustration or aversion, practice self-compassion instead. Continue your formal practice, and take some time to write in your journal about your experience of the practices so far, as well as any barriers you can identify.

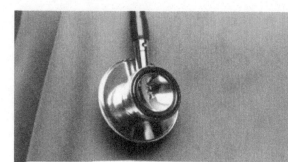

Points to Remember

+ Technology plays a significant role in modern nursing.
+ Patients can be overlooked when monitors and screens dominate.
+ Mindful nurses manage to retain a human connection with patients, despite the presence of technology.
+ Mindfulness can help you cope with the constant disruption of alarms and other devices.
+ With intentional practice, beeps and alarms can prompt you to become aware, rather than get distracted.

CHAPTER TWENTY ONE

Bringing Mindfulness and Compassion to Your Healthcare Facility

When we make a decision to honor our inner peace and allow it to blossom, we feel drawn to create peace in our external environment.

—Christopher Dines

Stacy Hayes was the director of nursing for a five hundred-bed city hospital. Although she didn't have the opportunity to take care of patients directly anymore, she was determined to make staff wellness a top priority. Her nurses kept quitting to take other jobs, and the nurses that remained faced shift after shift of short staffing. Alarmingly, it wouldn't be long before almost one third of Stacy's nursing staff had moved on because the work was so stressful.

While Stacy was attending an out-of-town convention, her attention was drawn to a booth that focused specifically on nurse wellness. The company offered resources to help staff cope with stress and burnout. Much of the information was centered on mindfulness training and promised that hospitals offering this would have healthier staff, less burnout, and less turnover.

At her wits' end, Stacy decided to give it a shot. On her return to the hospital, she distributed the information to raise awareness of mindfulness and recruited an experienced teacher to facilitate the sessions.

Following the training, Stacy surveyed the nurses to see if their stress levels had changed. Some nurses had not taken the training—they were skeptical and felt it wasn't for them—but most embraced the initiative and gave positive feedback. As the year progressed and trainings continued, Stacy found that her retention of nurses improved. She made mindfulness part of the annual training offered to nurses, and all new nurses who were interested were instructed in the basics.

As a result, a nurse approached Stacy at one of the trainings and thanked her. He told her that he had been on the verge of quitting nursing because the stress was getting to him. Luckily, mindfulness gave him a new lease on life and a sense of hope that he could weather whatever storms came his way. In the end, Stacy's emphasis on mindfulness reduced stress levels throughout the hospital—and Stacy herself benefited because she no longer had to constantly recruit new staff to replace all the nurses who were leaving.

Consider This:

Are your coworkers stressed out and unhappy? Are many of them quitting? Are you afraid that it will be too difficult and time-consuming to implement change? Do you feel it is in the nature of healthcare to be stressful and that nurses just need to learn to deal with it? Or do you feel nurses and other healthcare professionals are already compassionate as part of their job, and that training in this area is not necessary?

Imagine a workplace anchored in calm, no matter what pressures and demands the day might bring. Picture an environment forged in mutual harmony and unified intent, a place focused on comprehensive well-being. For the moment, imagine a mindful workplace.

Although mindfulness does not eliminate the challenges and chaos you deal with in the workplace, it can alter how you meet and respond to such challenges. Psychological well-being enhances productivity and success at work. In other words, the happier you are, the better your chances are to deliver your very best. Thanks to exhaustive research conducted over the last two decades, organizations are redefining their work environments and staff expectations. In particular, they no longer dismiss stress as an unavoidable side effect of the job, but regard it as a manageable parameter that can be reduced through careful interventions.

We know that happy staff enjoy the job and perform better.[71] Won over by the simplicity and efficiency of mindfulness, many workplaces across the globe, from giants like Google to family-run businesses, are taking note. From Apple to Ford, from Deutsche Bank to Starbucks, workplaces are introducing mindfulness with the goal to make their work environment happier and healthier for everyone. Patricia Reid Ponte, CNO at Boston's Dana-Farber Cancer Institute, believes that nursing should follow suit. "Nurse leaders in education and practice should move to recognize and integrate mindfulness-based practice as a core competency that supports effective nursing practice and therapeutic relationships with patients and families."[72]

Isn't it time you brought mindfulness to your healthcare facility?

Benefits of Mindfulness and Compassion in the Workplace

Being happy at work is possible for all of us, anytime and anywhere, with open eyes and a caring heart.

—Sharon Salzberg

Mindfulness and compassion are good practices for anyone and everyone. As you continue to practice them at work, not only will your enthusiasm for them grow as you witness the very real enhancements to the level of care you can now give, but also your coworkers will see the difference in you and how you relate to your patients and colleagues. What's more, your coworkers' interest offers an ideal opportunity to share your enthusiasm for these practices.

From physicians, nurses, psychologists, and midwives to administrators, general staff, and senior management, mindfulness is relevant at every rung of your organizational ladder. Whether you seek to improve working relationships, inspire better leadership, or promote mental well-being and stability during change, mindfulness is a skill and a practice that can transform healthcare. As you become mindful, you may become better able to advocate for change within your workplace, in relation to unfair conditions such as unsafe staffing levels, job insecurity, heavy workloads, increased patient acuity and numbers, technological change, and unfair pay practices.

Introducing Mindfulness to Your Workplace

If you feel inspired to introduce mindfulness to your workplace, remember that introducing a new practice or idea in a work environment presents challenges. For one thing, it means enlisting the help and cooperation of many busy, overworked professionals, and asking them to be a part of something that will likely change the way they see themselves, their work, and their patients. A quick tour through the proven benefits of mindfulness to both the individual and the organization can form a winning argument.

Year after year, stress affects not only employees but also the organizations that employ them. The National Institute for Occupational Safety and Health estimates that in the United States alone, stress-related ailments cost companies approximately two hundred billion dollars annually in absenteeism, workforce turnover, lowered productivity, and medical bills.[73] For everyone from general staff to CEOs, the adverse effects of long hours and workplace stress are reaching a critical climax.

Companies are now spending considerable resources on integrating mindfulness into wellness programs that train employees to actively handle stress. Corporate attention to the subject is making mindfulness more than just a buzzword in the modern workplace.

Mindfulness-Based Stress Reduction (MBSR) in Your Workplace

With the support of management, you can introduce MBSR at your healthcare facility by hiring a trainer to run the course in-house and making it available to staff at all levels. MBSR is the gold standard training in mindfulness, with an abundance of research citing its benefits. More than twenty thousand people have graduated from the program taught at the University of Massachusetts Medical Center.[74] Currently more than two hundred fifty clinics in the United States offer MBSR to their patients, and countless other clinical programs utilize mindfulness-based treatment approaches.[75] The popularity of mindfulness training increases yearly.

Basic MBSR

At the core of MBSR is an intensive training in mindfulness. MBSR consists of eight weekly two-and-a-half to three-hour sessions and includes forty-five minutes of daily home practice—also a daylong retreat between the sixth and seventh weeks. Each of the eight sessions has a central theme which is explored through practices, instruction, group discussion, and reflection. Sessions focus on cultivating the informal aspects of mindfulness to help participants integrate it into their daily lives. This format allows for regular check-ins between the tutor and participants and allows participation with steady momentum and involvement.[76]

If this schedule is not feasible for your facility, the course can also be adapted to the demands of your workplace and its schedules. For example, the eight-week course can be offered as a half-day session once every two weeks, for a period of sixteen weeks. Keep in mind that while half-day sessions may be easier to integrate into your workplace, the reduced frequency of meeting might weaken the integrity of the MBSR model (since motivation for regular home practice in the longer gap between sessions could be harder for students to sustain).

If your workforce or management is not yet ready to commit to a full MBSR program, you could introduce a series of shorter initiatives to stimulate interest and afford workers the opportunity to explore the practice at whatever level they *can* engage.

Issues and Desired Outcomes

MBSR can also be adapted to focus on specific health issues such as cancer or diabetes and to improve working relationships, general well-being, focus, and performance.

At the outset, it's important to identify clear outcomes for your program to allow clear and focused training as well as post-training evaluation. Doing so helps you choose the optimal instructor for your workplace by evaluating their skills and experience in light of your aims. Meet with your colleagues, hold discussions, or carry out quick surveys to identify which areas need focus at your facility.

Target Audience

Another important aspect to consider when organizing your training is the audience. Which group of colleagues will you target? Since MBSR can be applied at every level of your workplace, you could offer it to a focused group of staff who work closely with each other or to a mixed group from different departments.

Each group of people will be different. Some will have comfortable group dynamics, while others will have participants who will feel less able to express themselves freely. For that reason, you will have to organize your target participants with attention to how well certain professions mix, or based on their shared work environment or shared patient population. You can also organize one-on-one MBSR training, which may be a preferred option for senior management.

Evaluation

Instead of attempting to assess the effectiveness of MBSR in retrospect, work with your mindfulness instructor to establish clear evaluation procedures at the outset. Using your identified outcomes as a guide, work together to conduct surveys, collect and collate data, and create a clear vision of the desired training experience and facility goals. Bear in mind that pre-training polls and surveys also go a long way in shaping the format and structure of the course you organize.

Measures can include the Mindful Attention Awareness Scale, which you completed in Chapter 1. Presently, this handy tool is in the public domain and can be used freely for clinical or research purposes.

Other leading measurement tools include the Perceived Stress Scale to measure the perception of stress,[77] the Maslach Burnout Inventory to measure burnout,[78] and the Self-Compassion Scale to measure self-compassion.[79]

Recruiting a Course Instructor

A good course instructor must have extensive personal practice experience as well as theoretical learning. Further, a skilled instructor is not just proficient at delivering the training syllabus, but should also be able to adapt it to individual needs and environments.

If any nurses in your organization are certified in mindfulness training, they might be willing, even eager, to help you to facilitate MBSR. At present there are no mandatory requirements for mindfulness instructors, making it vital to do your homework to ensure you choose a knowledgeable, skilled, and well-trained facilitator. Fortunately, that's not as daunting as it sounds. The Center for Mindfulness at University of Massachusetts Medical School provides information relating to best-practice guidelines for trainers in the United States, and in the United Kingdom, the Network of Mindfulness-Based Teacher Training Organizations provides information, listings, and best-practice guidelines.

Here's a suggested checklist to use when choosing a workplace instructor:

- ☐ Verify the instructor's credentials—completion of a recognized teacher-training course based on MBSR or a similar course is essential.
- ☐ Make sure your instructor has a good foundation in mindfulness practice; a trainer should have practiced mindfulness for at least one to two years.
- ☐ Ideally your facilitator should have a professional background in mental health so that they can respond appropriately to any psychological issues experienced by participants during training.
- ☐ Make sure your instructor has some knowledge of your organization and its specific demands and challenges.
- ☐ Your instructor should engage actively and consistently in supervision sessions with suitably experienced mindfulness trainers or trainer networks as part of their continuing professional development.

Recruiting Participants

Championing the introduction of mindfulness-based practices in your workplace may require that you campaign for it. Following that, you might also have to advertise and promote the course to your colleagues.

Whether participation is voluntary or compulsory, informed participants are bound to be more enthusiastic and engaged. A good way to begin the process is by initiating an open discussion in your workplace. Are people familiar with mindfulness at any level? Have they practiced it or known anyone who does?

At first, some staff may resist engaging with mindfulness training as it might conjure up images of incense, robes, and chanting! Hear people out before gently dispelling any misconceived beliefs they may have.

Here are a few simple steps you can take to inform people:

- Distribute literature on MBSR and cite research showing the many benefits of this program (see the list of references and additional resources at the end of this book).
- Include a clear Outcome Statement in your promotional literature outlining what participants can anticipate from the course you plan to run.
- Team up with like-minded individuals in your workplace to establish a network of mindfulness champions—people are more likely to respond to those colleagues with whom they work most closely.

Shorter Mindfulness Programs

At present, your workforce or management may not yet be ready to commit to the full eight-week MBSR program. If that's the case, it's okay. As an option, you might introduce a series of shorter initiatives to stimulate interest and afford workers the opportunity to explore the practice at their own pace. Once you enlist the support of management, try doing the following at your healthcare facility:

- Organize hour-long "taster sessions" that workers can access during lunch or outside work hours.
- Incorporate mindfulness into other personal development initiatives, such as creativity training, stress management, resilience training, and emotional intelligence classes.
- Introduce the practice of "a mindfulness minute" at the beginning or end of each shift or at team meetings.
- Designate a corner or space in your facility as the "mindfulness area" to be used for quiet time and reflection.
- Conduct workshops on mindful leadership—how to lead with courage, compassion, and focus.
- Host both one-on-one and group sessions where employees can meditate alone or with others.
- Organize mindful walks outside the facility during lunch hours or after work.
- Share articles, research, and publications on mindfulness and its benefits.

Mindfulness for Patients

Without doubt, mindfulness is as beneficial for patients as it is for healthcare workers. A vital self-care tool, mindfulness is now gaining popularity as part of patients' post-discharge and long-term wellness plans.[80]

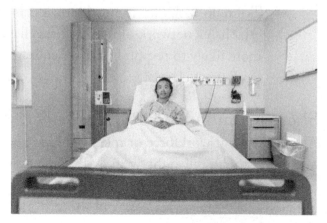

In order to be effective, before you start teaching it to your patients, mindfulness should be an integral part of your own life. In addition to the value of practicing what you preach, this is important for three reasons:

- 🌿 When you practice regularly, you gain a deeper understanding of the process.
- 🌿 You can more easily recognize whether mindfulness is appropriate for a particular patient.
- 🌿 Personal practice helps you to appreciate the varying challenges people face in modifying their deep-seated conditioning.

Journal Reflection:

What in your experience is changing as you continue your daily mindfulness and compassion practice?

What challenges do you face in sustaining your daily practice?

How open is your healthcare facility to mindfulness and compassion training for staff and/or patients?

What role, if any, could you play in this initiative?

Without nurses themselves learning to practice and integrate mindfulness into their own lives, they will be unable, skillfully, to offer it as a holistic practice and perspective to those health populations they serve. Placing attention on how to integrate mindfulness into nursing education and practice would strengthen their ability to offer this knowledge to others.

—Lacie White

How to Strengthen Compassion in Your Workplace

Recent research suggests that workers are happier, more efficient, and less stressed in a compassionate workplace.[81] That makes a strong business case for compassion training at an organizational level. In light of these findings, how can you strengthen compassion levels in your workplace so that everyone benefits?

Promoting compassion in one's healthcare facility is a three-pronged endeavor. First, staff should receive formal training and education in the meaning and practice of compassion. Second, numerous steps should be introduced to create awareness and facilitate a more compassionate workplace. Third, a facility-wide initiative can be developed to prevent, identify, and treat compassion fatigue among healthcare workers.

Promoting Compassion in Healthcare Facilities Requires:
- Training and education focused on compassion
- Developing a compassionate workplace
- Addressing compassion fatigue

To this end, you can introduce formal training programs at your facility to strengthen compassion in staff. Of course, workplace training can happen only with sufficient funding and the buy-in of your organization's senior management, but there are several training options available to suit all budgets. For example, staff members can be invited to participate in a formal compassion-training program with occasional refresher retraining. This can be offered as a part of skills development and performance management. Less formal measures can also be introduced to promote awareness of the importance of compassion in the workplace. These programs form the basis for understanding how important compassion is and how to practice it, beginning with oneself.

The Compassion Cultivation Training Program

Perhaps the best known and most widely used compassion training program available, Compassion Cultivation Training (CCT) is a nine-week standardized program developed by the Stanford University Center for Compassion and Altruism Research and Education.[82] The program consists of a two-hour weekly class with homework assignments. During the program, participants are encouraged to practice meditation for at least fifteen minutes daily to develop loving-kindness, empathy, and compassion.

You can help make compassion training available to staff members by hiring a qualified trainer to deliver the course. Most facilities hire external trainers, but some facilities are fortunate enough to already have qualified trainers on staff.

CCT can help healthcare workers to strengthen compassion levels and develop the resilience needed to cope with distress in themselves and others. Further, it can help staff to prevent or recover from compassion fatigue. Research to date shows that CCT reduces worry and mind wandering, and engenders significant improvements in compassion for others, from others, and for oneself.[83, 84, 85]

Other Programs for Compassion Training

Two other excellent programs for compassion training are The Mindful Self Compassion Program (www.self-compassion.org), and the Cognitively-Based Compassion Training (www.tibet.emory.edu/cognitively-based-compassion-training). Schwartz Center Rounds also build compassion by focusing on the emotions, challenges, stresses and interpersonal dynamics of caregiving.

Developed in 1994 at the Schwartz Center for Compassionate Healthcare in Boston, Schwartz Center Rounds have been implemented in more than three hundred fifty healthcare facilities in the United States.[86] Sessions are scheduled once a month for an hour over breakfast or lunch. During that time, clinical and nonclinical staff from all organizational levels explore the impact that work and patients have on their emotions and quality of life. Each individual has the opportunity to tell their stories and share their experiences, which everyone present can then reflect on and explore.

Typically, rounds begin with a brief presentation of a patient case and a selected psychosocial topic. Then a facilitated discussion follows, wherein caregivers from diverse disciplines reflect on the emotional challenges of patient care.[87] As such, the program provides a dedicated time to freely and safely share difficult feelings, such as anger, guilt, sadness, and frustration as well as an opportunity to express feelings of joy, gratitude, and pride.

In the United Kingdom, Schwartz Center Rounds are currently available in eighty hospitals and hospices.[88] Generally, a multidisciplinary team led by a senior doctor sponsored by the organization's executive board organizes the rounds, which are attended by twenty to two hundred people at a time.[89]

Retrospective surveys have found benefits of Schwartz Center Rounds include increased awareness of the importance of empathy, better teamwork, appreciation for colleagues' contributions, decreased stress, improved ability to cope, positive changes in institutional culture, better relationships among caregivers and patients, and heightened awareness of self-care.[90] A study of English hospitals over a one-year, ten-round pilot period attended by twelve hundred fifty staff, found that Schwartz Center Rounds resulted in patient benefits and better teamwork.[91]

Obviously, bringing the mindfulness revolution and compassion training to your workplace can present a significant challenge. This type of system-wide change requires commitment, patience, efficient planning, and organization. You may meet resistance, delays, and unforeseen challenges, but the difficulties you face are worth enduring for the rewards of a workforce guided by mindfulness and compassion.

Practice Plan:

If reading this book was the first step on your mindfulness journey, congratulations! You have reached the end of your beginning. Take some time now to reflect on what you got from the practices

described here, as well as your intentions going forward
you learned? What will you bring with you as you mo\
Sustain your formal daily practice, choosing any combination
practices you explored in this book. Remember, too, that your life
is your practice—every moment offers an opportunity to cultivate
mindfulness and compassion. May you seize every moment!

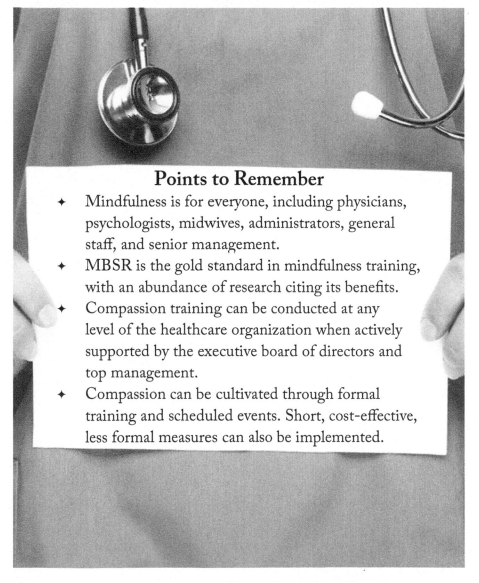

Points to Remember

+ Mindfulness is for everyone, including physicians, psychologists, midwives, administrators, general staff, and senior management.
+ MBSR is the gold standard in mindfulness training, with an abundance of research citing its benefits.
+ Compassion training can be conducted at any level of the healthcare organization when actively supported by the executive board of directors and top management.
+ Compassion can be cultivated through formal training and scheduled events. Short, cost-effective, less formal measures can also be implemented.

Moving Forward Mindfully

Researchers have studied and substantiated the benefits of mindfulness and compassion. Anchored in ancient wisdom and modern research, these practices span time, tradition, and culture to offer a comprehensive approach to managing well-being. Studies clearly show that they help fortify individual and collective well-being in the workplace.

Day in and day out, you and your fellow nurses are tasked with enormous responsibility. Given the pressures of your work, you may be hard-pressed to find a minute of spare time to focus on your own well-being, but it is well worth the effort to do so. Even short moments of daily mindfulness and compassion practice can profoundly affect you, your colleagues, and your work environment.

I hope this book has led you to experience some of the many benefits that mindfulness has to offer. I encourage you to continue using these practices to nurture the growth of mindfulness and compassion in your life. If you have found it helpful to read this information, consider taking a course to develop your practice further.

Keep in mind that mindfulness is a way of life, not simply a set of techniques. Even the briefest moments of practice do make a difference. Through them, your mindfulness muscle will grow stronger and your compassionate presence will deepen. Practice patiently going forward, being open to whatever unfolds, trusting in your own innate capacity for presence and well-being.

May you be well, and may your practice touch the lives of others deeply! In closing, I would like to share the following excerpt from a poem by John O' Donohue:

For a Nurse

May you embrace the beauty in what you do
and how you stand like a secret angel
between the bleak despair of illness
and the unquenchable light of spirit
that can turn the darkest destiny toward dawn.

May you never doubt the gifts you bring
rather, learn from these frontiers
wisdom for your own heart.
May you come to inherit
the blessings of your kindness
and never be without care and love
when winter enters your own life.

—John O' Donohue

Appendix A: List of Practices

Use this handy list as a reminder of the practices you learned in this book. Each practice helps you to come off autopilot and bring your attention into the present moment.

Mindfulness in a Moment

The 3 Ps 54
Three-Step Breathing Space 83
STOP Practice...... 280
Two Feet, One Breath.. 284
Mindfulness Bell 304

Sitting Meditation

Mindful Breathing Practice..................................... 39
Awareness of Emotions in the Body 121
Observing Thoughts 238
Open-Awareness Meditation 265

Mindfulness of the Body

Mindful Steps... 94
Mindful Balance 95
Mindful Foot care 98
Mindful Check-in 105
Mindful Hands 107
Body Scan..... 109
Short Body Scan...... 113
Mindfulness of Sounds... 115
Informal Walking Meditation.................................. 118
Formal Walking Meditation 119
Being in Your Body.. 130
Exploring Difficult Sensations 137

Mindfulness of Difficult Sensations 140
Respond Mindfully to Stress 154

Mindful Movement
Mindful Lifting 131
Seated Poses 163
Standing Poses 165

Mindfulness of Everyday Activities
Mindful Eating.. 62
Mindful Handwashing 64
Mindful Daily Activities....................................... 92
Mindful Reflection 274
Mindful Medication Administration 275
Handover Reflection 291
Mindful Use of Computers 302

Compassion Practices
GRACE Practice.......... 183
Self-Compassion Break.. 208
Compassionate Letter Writing................................. 209
Loving-Kindness Meditation 216
Loving-Kindness Meditation for Caregivers..................... 219
Just Like Me... 223
Tonglen-on-the-Spot... 227
Compassion Mantra.. 229
Compassion Reflection 230

Interpersonal Mindfulness
Mindful Speech... 256
Mindful Listening 263
Mindful Presence 49
Mindful Interaction... 278
Mindful Encounter 301

Appendix B: ProQOL

PROFESSIONAL QUALITY OF LIFE SCALE (PROQOL)
COMPASSION SATISFACTION AND COMPASSION FATIGUE
(PROQOL) VERSION 5 (2009)

When you nurse people you have direct contact with their lives. As you may have found, your compassion for those you nurse can affect you in positive and negative ways. Below are some questions about your experiences, both positive and negative, as a nurse. Consider each of the following questions about you and your current work situation. Select the number that honestly reflects how frequently you experienced these things in the last 30 days.

| 1=Never | 2=Rarely | 3=Sometimes | 4=Often | 5=Very Often |

_____ 1. I am happy.
_____ 2. I am preoccupied with more than one person I nurse.
_____ 3. I get satisfaction from being able to nurse people.
_____ 4. I feel connected to others.
_____ 5. I jump or am startled by unexpected sounds.
_____ 6. I feel invigorated after working with those I nurse.
_____ 7. I find it difficult to separate my personal life from my life as a nurse.
_____ 8. I am not as productive at work because I am losing sleep over traumatic experiences of a person I nurse.
_____ 9. I think that I might have been affected by the traumatic stress of those I nurse.
_____ 10. I feel trapped by my job as a nurse.
_____ 11. Because of my nursing, I have felt "on edge" about various things.
_____ 12. I like my work as a nurse.
_____ 13. I feel depressed because of the traumatic experiences of the people I nurse.
_____ 14. I feel as though I am experiencing the trauma of someone I have nursed.
_____ 15. I have beliefs that sustain me.
_____ 16. I am pleased with how I am able to keep up with nursing techniques and protocols.
_____ 17. I am the person I always wanted to be.
_____ 18. My work makes me feel satisfied.
_____ 19. I feel worn out because of my work as a nurse.
_____ 20. I have happy thoughts and feelings about those I nurse and how I could help them.
_____ 21. I feel overwhelmed because my patient load seems endless.
_____ 22. I believe I can make a difference through my work.
_____ 23. I avoid certain activities or situations because they remind me of frightening experiences of the people I nurse.
_____ 24. I am proud of what I can do to nurse.
_____ 25. As a result of my nursing, I have intrusive, frightening thoughts.
_____ 26. I feel "bogged down" by the system.
_____ 27. I have thoughts that I am a "success" as a nurse.
_____ 28. I can't recall important parts of my work with trauma victims.
_____ 29. I am a very caring person.
_____ 30. I am happy that I chose to do this work.

YOUR SCORES ON THE PROQOL: PROFESSIONAL QUALITY OF LIFE SCREENING

Based on your responses, place your personal scores below. If you have any concerns, you should discuss them with a physical or mental health care professional.

Compassion Satisfaction _____

Compassion satisfaction is about the pleasure you derive from being able to do your work well. For example, you may feel like it is a pleasure to help others through your work. You may feel positively about your colleagues or your ability to contribute to the work setting or even the greater good of society. Higher scores on this scale represent a greater satisfaction related to your ability to be an effective caregiver in your job.

The average score is 50 (SD 10; alpha scale reliability .88). About 25% of people score higher than 57 and about 25% of people score below 43. If you are in the higher range, you probably derive a good deal of professional satisfaction from your position. If your scores are below 40, you may either find problems with your job, or there may be some other reason—for example, you might derive your satisfaction from activities other than your job.

Burnout _____

Most people have an intuitive idea of what burnout is. From the research perspective, burnout is one of the elements of Compassion Fatigue (CF). It is associated with feelings of hopelessness and difficulties in dealing with work or in doing your job effectively. These negative feelings usually have a gradual onset. They can reflect the feeling that your efforts make no difference, or they can be associated with a very high workload or a non-supportive work environment. Higher scores on this scale mean that you are at higher risk for burnout.

The average score on the burnout scale is 50 (SD 10; alpha scale reliability .75). About 25% of people score above 57 and about 25% of people score below 43. If your score is below 43, this probably reflects positive feelings about your ability to be effective in your work. If you score above 57 you may wish to think about what at work makes you feel like you are not effective in your position. Your score may reflect your mood; perhaps you were having a "bad day" or are in need of some time off. If the high score persists or if it is reflective of other worries, it may be a cause for concern.

Secondary Traumatic Stress _____

The second component of Compassion Fatigue (CF) is secondary traumatic stress (STS). It is about your work related, secondary exposure to extremely or traumatically stressful events. Developing problems due to exposure to other's trauma is somewhat rare but does happen to many people who care for those who have experienced extremely or traumatically stressful events. For example, you may repeatedly hear stories about the traumatic things that happen to other people, commonly called Vicarious Traumatization. If your work puts you directly in the path of danger, for example, field work in a war or area of civil violence, this is not secondary exposure; your exposure is primary. However, if you are exposed to others' traumatic events as a result of your work, for example, as a therapist or an emergency worker, this is secondary exposure. The symptoms of STS are usually rapid in onset and associated with a particular event. They may include being afraid, having difficulty sleeping, having images of the upsetting event pop into your mind, or avoiding things that remind you of the event.

The average score on this scale is 50 (SD 10; alpha scale reliability .81). About 25% of people score below 43 and about 25% of people score above 57. If your score is above 57, you may want to take some time to think about what at work may be frightening to you or if there is some other reason for the elevated score. While higher scores do not mean that you do have a problem, they are an indication that you may want to examine how you feel about your work and your work environment. You may wish to discuss this with your supervisor, a colleague, or a health care professional.

WHAT IS MY SCORE AND WHAT DOES IT MEAN?

In this section, you will score your test so you understand the interpretation for you. To find your score on each section, total the questions listed on the left and then find your score in the table on the right of the section.

Compassion Satisfaction Scale

Copy your rating on each of these questions on to this table and add them up. When you have added them up you can find your score on the table to the right.

3. ____
6. ____
12. ____
16. ____
18. ____
20. ____
22. ____
24. ____
27. ____
30. ____

Total: _____

The sum of my Compassion Satisfaction questions is	So my Score Equals	And my Compassion Satisfaction level is
22 or less	43 or less	Low
Between 23 and 41	Around 50	Average
42 or more	57 or more	High

Burnout Scale

On the burnout scale you will need to take an extra step. Starred items are "reverse scored." If you scored the item 1, write a 5 beside it. The reason we ask you to reverse the scores is because scientifically the measure works better when these questions are asked in a positive way though they can tell us more about their negative form. For example, question 1. "I am happy" tells us more about the effects of helping when you are not happy so you reverse the score.

*1. ____ = ____
*4. ____ = ____
8. ____
10. ____
*15. ____ = ____
*17. ____ = ____
19. ____
21. ____
26. ____
*29. ____ = ____

Total: _____

The sum of my Burnout Questions is	So my Score Equals	And my Burnout level is
22 or less	43 or less	Low
Between 23 and 41	Around 50	Average
42 or more	57 or more	High

You Wrote	Change to
1	5
2	4
3	3
4	2
5	1

Secondary Traumatic Stress Scale

Just as you did on Compassion Satisfaction, copy your rating on each of these questions on to this table and add them up. When you have added them up you can find your score on the table to the right.

2. ____
5. ____
7. ____
9. ____
11. ____
13. ____
14. ____
23. ____
25. ____
28. ____

Total: _____

The sum of my Secondary Trauma questions is	So my Score Equals	And my Secondary Traumatic Stress level is
22 or less	43 or less	Low
Between 23 and 41	Around 50	Average
42 or more	57 or more	High

Additional Resources (by Chapter)

Chapter 1

Bring Mindfulness into Your Day. This article outlines several ways to inspire you to bring mindfulness into your day wherever you are. www.actionforhappiness.org/take-action/bring-mindfulness-into-your-day.

Chapter 2

The Mindfulness Bell rings periodically during the day to give you the opportunity to come off autopilot, check in for a moment, and notice what you are currently doing and in what state of mind you are while you are doing it. The app is available from https://play.google.com.

To listen to mindfulness audios recorded by Jon Kabat-Zinn, visit www.mindfulnesscds.com.

Chapter 3

Healing and the Mind: Healing from Within. This video documentary released by Bill Moyers in 1993 explores alternative approaches to medicine. The first half of the video shows Jon Kabat-Zinn leading participants through the eight-week MBSR class. Watching the video is a good way to get a feel for the eight-week course and how it can make a difference in people's lives. When first released, millions in the United States watched this documentary, which generated a huge interest in mindfulness. https://vimeo.com/39767361.

Chapter 4

Mindful.org. This information-packed website has news, updates, and articles on all aspects of mindfulness. Mindful.org also publishes the monthly *Mindful* magazine as well personal stories, news-you-can-use, advice, and insights.

Chapter 5

Nursing Blogs. In their excellent nursing blogs, Amanda Anderson *(thisnursewonders.com)* and Kateri Allard *(accordingtokateri.com)* often address issues relating to self-care. Nurse Keith, an award-winning blogger, hosts a popular nursing blog called "Digital Doorway." He also offers coaching for nurses—focusing on burnout prevention and recovery—under the auspices of NurseKeith.com and http://digitaldoorway.blogspot.ie/.

Chapter 6

Walking Meditation. Three walking meditations are available from Meditation Oasis as an MP3 and a smart phone app on Apple and Android phones. Each meditation has a slightly different focus: Being Fully Present, Enlivening the Body, and Enhancing the Senses. www.meditationoasis.com

Chapter 7

Looking after Your Health: Avoiding Back Injury, by Sara Randall, examines how to maintain back health in healthcare professionals—particularly midwives—and prevent injury through principles of good practice. Source: *The Practising Midwife,* Volume 17, Number 11, December 2014, pp. 10-14(5), Publisher: Medical Education Solutions Limited.
Hospitals Fail to Protect Nursing Staff from Becoming Patients: NPR Investigates. NPR news ran a multi-week series of stories on injury among nurses in February 2015. http://wgbhnews.org/post/hospitals-fail-protect-nursing-staff-becoming-patients

Chapter 8

In *Mindfulness for Pain Relief: Guided Practices for Reclaiming Your Body and Your Life,* Jon Kabat-Zinn leads guided meditations drawn from MBSR to help work with and find relief from chronic and acute pain, everyday stress, and emotional challenges. Audio program available from: SoundsTrue.com and Amazon.com.

The Back Sense Program for Treating Chronic Pain, by Ron Siegel, presents a treatment approach for chronic back pain based on scientific advances that show most chronic back pain is caused by stress, fear, muscle tension, and inactivity rather than by damage to the spine. For details, visit www.backsense.org.

Breathworks offers Mindfulness-Based Pain Management (MBPM) for people living with chronic pain. Although similar to MBSR and MBCT, MBPM has some specific applications for people living with pain and illness. These include a distinctive approach to mindfulness in daily life and mindful movement. Breathworks MBPM also includes compassion and acceptance meditations as part of the core curriculum. For details, visit http://www.breathworks-mindfulness.org.uk

Chapter 9

The Mindfulness App helps you train yourself in mindfulness wherever you are and cope with everyday stress. A team of Dutch psychologists who are also recognized and experienced mindfulness trainers developed the app. For details or to download, visit http://www.mindfulness-app.com/.

Chapter 10

Yoga Nursing is a new movement in healthcare, nursing, and yoga created by Annette Tersigni, a holistic RN, stress-relief expert, back-safety expert, and medical yoga therapist. Yoga Nursing unites the ancient wisdom of yoga with the modern science of nursing. Its mission is to train and create "yoga nurses" to support the ailing healthcare system and relieve stress, anxiety, pain, and suffering for both nurses and their patients. www.yoganurse.com Anne Cushman's book, *Moving into Meditation: A 12-Week Mindfulness Program for Yoga Practitioners*, is an excellent guide to cultivating a mindful relationship with your body by blending yoga and mindfulness meditation. For information on her retreats, classes, and online courses, visit http://annecushman.com/.

Chapter 11

The *Greater Good Science Center* at the University of California, Berkeley researches the sociology, psychology, and neuroscience of well-being and teaches skills that foster a resilient and compassionate society. The website offers many free and downloadable articles on compassion and mindfulness. http://greatergood.berkeley.edu/

Chapter 12

Hearts in Healthcare focuses on the critical importance of compassion in healthcare. Founded by Robin Youngson, this site is a hub where you can find articles, inspiration, resources, and campaigns focusing on compassion in healthcare as well as information about Robin's excellent book, *Time to Care*. http://heartsinhealthcare.com/

Workshops for Helping Professions. Françoise Mathieu is director of Compassion Fatigue Solutions, which offers training to helpers on topics related to self-care, wellness, burnout, and compassion fatigue. For details, visit www.compassionfatigue.ca.

Patricia Smith is founder of the Compassion Fatigue Awareness Project and Healthy Caregiving, LLC, which offer workshops, training materials, and workbooks. For information, visit www.compassionfatigue.org and http://www.healthycaregiving.com/.

Chapter 13

Audio Resources for Cultivating Compassion

The following three websites offer excellent self-compassion practices freely available as downloads:

Dr. Chris Germer, author of *The Mindful Path to Self-Compassion*, offers several meditations on this site to guide you through the first phase of mindful self-compassion training. www.mindfulselfcompassion.org

Kristin Neff's website offers several valuable compassion practices for download in both audio and text. http://www.self-compassion.org

Professor *Paul Gilbert* offers a selection of valuable audio files from his Compassionate Mind Training. Practices offered include Soothing Rhythm Breathing, Compassionate Self-Imagery, and Our Ideal Compassionate Other. www.compassionatemind.co.uk

Chapter 14

Sharon Salzberg, one of the first teachers to bring loving-kindness meditation to the West, is a founding member of this Yahoo group that offers a place for you to share your experiences with meditation and loving-kindness meditation and to express insights, ask questions, and most importantly, lend support to one another in your practice. https://groups.yahoo.com/neo/groups/giftoflovingkindness/info

Chapter 15

The *Get Self-Help* website offers excellent Cognitive Behavior Therapy (CBT) information, resources, and worksheets freely available for download. http://www.getselfhelp.co.uk

Chapter 16

Thich Nhat Hanh's book, *Work*, has many practices relevant for cultivating harmony in work teams. Publisher: Parallax Press, Feb. 2013.

Chapter 17

Insight Dialogue is an interpersonal meditation practice that brings the mindfulness and tranquility of silent meditation directly into your experiences with other people. Gregory Kramer, the founder of Insight Dialogue, describes how the practice is accessible for meditators and non-meditators alike and can serve as a pathway for people to encounter a felt sense of what is like to be with others and be with oneself in awareness and receptivity. www.metta.org

Chapter 18

Can Mindfulness Prevent Potentially Hazardous Errors? This article shares tips for staying focused on the task and avoiding serious mistakes. http://safety.blr.com/workplace-safety-news/safety-administration/safety-general/Can-mindfulness-prevent-potentially-hazardous-erro/

Chapter 19

Five Tips for a Great Hand-Off Report. This short article is full of useful tips to ensure your handover is a success. http://scrubsmag.com/giving-a-good-report/

Chapter 20

Using Technology Mindfully. This useful article outlines tips to help you stay in control of technology as opposed to having technology control you. The tips can help you balance your relationship with your high-tech gadgets. http://mindfulhub.com/wp-content/uploads/Using-Technology-Mindfully-PR.pdf

Chapter 21

The Center for Compassion and Altruism Research and Education investigates methods to cultivate compassion within individuals and society. In addition, CCARE provides teacher training in their compassion-cultivation program, as well as educational public events and programs. Learn more at http://ccare.stanford.edu/about/mission-vision/#sthash.qU1400Yh.dpuf.

Professional MBSR Training. If you would like to bring mindfulness to your healthcare facility, you can train to become a mindfulness teacher. The following centers offer comprehensive professional training in teaching MBSR:

Mindfulness-Based Stress Reduction
Center for Mindfulness in Medicine, Health Care, and Society
222 Maple Ave, Shrewsbury, MA 01545
www.umassmed.edu/cfm

Centre for Mindfulness Research and Practice
School of Psychology
Dean St Building
Bangor University
Bangor LL57 1UT
United Kingdom
http://www.bangor.ac.uk/mindfulness/

Notes

1   Cathryn Domrose, "Meditation Offers Benefits for Nurses and Patients," *Nurse.com* June 6, 2010. http://news.nurse.com/article/20100606/ NATIONAL02/306060011/-1/frontpage#.VXH535VFDIU.

2   Jon Kabat-Zinn, *Wherever You Go, There You Are: Mindfulness Meditation in Everyday Life* (New York: Hyperion, 1994).

3   Kirk Warren Brown and Richard M. Ryan, "The Benefits of Being Present: Mindfulness and its Role in Psychological Well-Being," *Journal of Personality and Social Psychology* 84, no. 4 (2003): 822-48, doi:10.1037/0022-3514.84.4.822.

4   Kelley Raab, "Mindfulness, Self-Compassion, and Empathy among Health Care Professionals: A Review of the Literature," *Journal of Health Care Chaplaincy* 20, no. 3 (2014): 95-108, doi10.1080/08854726.2014.913876.

5   Britta K.Hölzel et al.,"Mindfulness Practice Leads to Increases in Regional Brain Gray Matter Density," *Psychiatry Research: Neuroimaging*191, no. 1 (2011): 36,doi:10.1016/j.pscychresns.2010.08.006.

6   Dacher Keltner, "We are Built to be Kind," Fig. 1, *University of California*, YouTube video, 4:36, posted December 2, 2014, https://www.youtube.com/ watch?v=SsWs6bf7t. https://www.youtube.com/watch?v=SsWs6bf7t.

7   Raab, "Mindfulness, Self-Compassion, and Empathy among Health Care Professionals."

8   Mary E. Wilbur, "Leading the Way: Zen at Work; The Use of Meditation in Nursing Practice," *Gastroenterology Nursing* 26, no. 4 (2003): 169.

9   Matthew A. Killingsworth and Daniel T. Gilbert, "A Wandering Mind is an Unhappy Mind," *Science* 330, no. 6006 (2010): 932, doi: 10.1126/ science.1192439.

10 University of Wisconsin Department of Family Medicine and Community Health, "1. Pause (Practice in Your Practice)," http://www.fammed.wisc.edu/ mindfulness/pip-pause/.

11 Christiane Wolf and Greg Serpa, *A Clinician's Guide to Teaching Mindfulness* (Oakland, CA: New Harbinger Publications, 2015).

12 Amanda Anderson, "The Poetry of the IV," *This Nurse Wonders*, September 16, 2014, http://thisnursewonders.com/2014/09/16/the-poetry-of-the-iv/.

13 Andrew Hafenbrack et al., "Debiasing the Mind Through Meditation: Mindfulness and the Sunk-Cost Bias," *Psychological Science* 25, no. 2 (2013) 369-76.

14 Mark Williams, John Teasdale, Zindel Segal, and Jon Kabat-Zinn, *The Mindful Way through Depression: Freeing Yourself from Chronic Unhappiness* (New York: Guilford Press, 2007).

15 David C. Holzman, "What's in a Color? The Unique Human Health Effects of Blue Light," *Environmental Health Perspectives* 118, no. 1 (2010): A22-A27, doi:10.1289/ehp.118-a22.

16 John O'Donohue, *To Bless the Space Between Us: A Book of Blessings* (USA: Doubleday, 2008).

17 Diann Neu, "Blessing Our Hands," adapted by Corlette Pierson from "In Praise of Hands" Waterwheel Winter (1989). The Women's Alliance for Theology, Ethics and Ritual, 8121 Georgia Avenue, Suite 310, Silver Spring, MD 20910 USA. www.waterwomensalliance.org, dneu@hers.com.

18 Ann Hendrich et al., "A 36-Hospital Time and Motion Study: How do Medical-Surgical Nurses Spend their Time?" *The Permanente Journal* 12, no. 3 (2008): 25-34.

19 US Department of Labor, Bureau of Labor Statistics, "Injuries, Illnesses, and Fatalities," last modified June 19, 2015, http://www.bls.gov/iif/oshfaq1.htm#q166.

20 Kate Kay and Nel Glass, "Debunking the Manual Handling Myth: An Investigation of Manual Handling Knowledge and Practices in the Australian Private Health Sector," *International Journal of Nursing Practice* 17 (2011): 231-37, doi:10.1111/j.1440-172x.2011.01930.x.

21 Kyung Ja June and Sung-Hyu Cho, "Low-Back Pain and Work-Related Factors Using Nurses in Intensive Care Units," *Journal of Clinical Nursing* 20, no. 3-4 (2011): 479-87, doi:10.1111/j.1365-2702.2010.03210.x.

22 Royal College of Nursing (RCN), *Good Practice for Handling Feedback* (London: Royal College of Nursing, 2014).

23 Pamela Gray-Toft and James G. Anderson, "The Nursing Stress Scale: Development of an Instrument," *Journal of Behavioral Assessment* 3, no. 1 (1981): 11-23, doi:10.1007/BF01321348.

24 Jon Kabat-Zinn, *Full Catastrophe Living: Using the Wisdom of your Body and Mind to Face Stress, Pain, and Illness* (New York: Dell Publishing, 1991).

25 Helen E. Tilbrook et al., "Yoga for Chronic Low Back Pain: A Randomized Trial," *Annals of Intern Medicine* 155 (2011): 569-78, doi:10.7326/0003-4819-155-9-201111010-00003.

[26] Paul Condon and David DeSteno, "Compassion for One Reduces Punishment for Another," *Journal of Experimental Social Psychology* 47 (2011): 698-701, doi:10.1016/j.jesp.2010.11.016.

[27] Marianna Diomidous et al., "Descriptive Study of Nursing Students' Motives to Choose Nursing as a Career," *Greek Journal of Nursing Science 2*, no. 5 (2013): 60-66.

[28] Dignity Health, "Scientific Literature Review Shows Health Care Delivered with Kindness and Compassion Leads to Faster Healing, Reduced Pain," press release, November 12, 2014, http://www.reuters.com/article/2014/11/12/ca-dignity-health-idUSnBw125352a+100+BSW20141112.

[29] Jill Shuman, "Enhancing Patient Adherence: And What to Do When All Else Fails," *Primary Care Network*, October 19, 2010, http://www.primaryissues.org/2010/10/enhancing-patient-adherence-and-what-to-do-when-all-else-fails.

[30] Sigal G. Barsade and Olivia A. O'Neill, "What's Love Got to Do with It? A Longitudinal Study of the Culture of Companionate Love and Employee and Client Outcomes in a Long-Term Care Setting," *Administrative Science Quarterly* 59, no. 4 (2014): 551-98, doi:10.1177/0001839214538636.

[31] Giuseppe Di Pellegrino, Luciano Fadiga, Leonardo Fogassi, Vittorio Gallese, & Giacomo Rizzolatti, "Understanding Motor Events: A Neurophysiological Study," *Experimental Brain Research 91*, no. 1 (1992): 176-180.

[32] Paul Condon, Gaëlle Desbordes, Willa B. Miller, and David DeSteno, "Meditation Increases Compassionate Responses to Suffering," *Psychological Science 24*, no. 10 (2013), doi: 10.1177/0956797613485603.

[33] Paul Gilbert, and Choden, *Mindful Compassion* (London: Constable Robinson, 2013).

[34] Joan Halifax, "G.R.A.C.E. for Nurses: Cultivating Compassion in Nurse/Patient Interactions," *Journal of Nursing Education and Practice 4*, no. 1 (2014): 121-28.

[35] Clara Joinson, "Coping with Compassion Fatigue," *Nursing* 22 (1992): 116-21.

[36] Christina S. Melvin, "Professional Compassion Fatigue: What is the True Cost of Nurses Caring for the Dying?" *International Journal of Palliative Nursing 18*, no. 12 (2012): 606-611.

[37] Françoise Mathieu, "Compassion Fatigue," in *Encyclopedia of Trauma: An Interdisciplinary Guide*, ed. Charles R. Figley, (Los Angeles: Sage Publications, 2012),136-39.

[38] American Psychiatric Association, *Diagnostic and Statistical Manual of Mental Disorders: DSM-V*, 5th ed. (Arlington, VA: Author, 2013).

[39] Deborah A. Boyle, "Countering Compassion Fatigue: A Requisite Nursing Agenda," *Online Journal of Issues in Nursing* 16, no. 1 (2011): 1, doi:10.3912/OJIN.Vol16No01Man02.

[40] Barbara Lombardo and Caryl Eyre, "Compassion Fatigue: A Nurse's Primer," *Online Journal of Issues in Nursing* 16, no. 1 (2011): 3, doi:10.3912/OJIN.Vol16No01Man03.

[41] B. Hudnall Stamm, "Professional Quality of Life: Compassion Satisfaction and Fatigue (ProQOL)," version 5, last modified 2009, http://www.proqol.org.

[42] Christie Lane, "Yoga and Mindfulness: Perspective of an RN Yoga Instructor," *Journal of Nursing, UC San Diego* (Summer 2014): 7-9, https://health.ucsd.edu/medinfo/nursing/Documents/Nursing-Sum-2014.pdf.

[43] Elizabeth A. Yoder, "Caring Too Much: Compassion Fatigue in Nursing," *Applied Nursing Research 23*, no. 4 (2010): 191-197.

[44] Kristin D. Neff, "The Development and Validation of a Scale to Measure Self-compassion," *Self and Identity* 2 (2003): 223-50, doi: 10.1080/15298860309027.

[45] Ibid.

[46] Laura K. Barnard and John F. Curry, "Self-Compassion: Conceptualizations, Correlates, & Interventions," *Review of General Psychology* 15, no. 4 (2011): 289–303.

[47] Kristin D. Neff and Christopher K. Germer, "A Pilot Study and Randomized Controlled Trial of the Mindful Self-compassion Program," *Journal of Clinical Psychology* 69 (2013): 28-44.

[48] Kristin Neff, http://self-compassion.org.

[49] Sharon Salzberg, *Real Happiness: The Power of Meditation: A 28-Day Program* (New York: Workman, 2011), p. 160.

[50] Emma M. Seppala et al.,"Loving-Kindness Meditation: A Tool to Improve Healthcare Provider Compassion, Resilience, and Patient Care," *Journal of Compassionate Healthcare* 1 (2014): 5, doi:10.1186/s40639-014-0005-9.

[51] Elizabeth A. Hoge et al., "Loving-Kindness Meditation Practice Associated with Longer Telomeres in Women," *Brain Behavior and Immunity* 32 (2013): 159-63, doi:10.1016/j.bbi.2013.04.0055.

52 James W. Carson et al., "Loving-Kindness Meditation for Chronic Low-Back Pain: Results from a Pilot Trial," *Journal of Holistic Nursing* 23, no. 3 (2005): 287-304, doi:10.1177/0898010105277651.

53 Ibid.

54 E.g., Hoge et al., "Loving-Kindness Meditation Practice"; Bethany E. Kok et al.,"How Positive Emotions Build Physical Health: Perceived Positive Social Connections Account for the Upward Spiral between Positive Emotions and Vagal Tone," *Psychological Science* 24, no. 7 (2013): 1123-32, doi:10.1177/0956797612470827; Makenzie E. Tonelli and Amy B. Wachholtz, "Meditation-based Treatment Yielding Immediate Relief for Meditation Naïve Migraineurs," *Pain Management Nursing* 15, no. 1 (2014): 36-40, doi:10.1016/j.pmn.2012.04.002.

55 Frank Jude Boccio, "Love in Full Bloom," *Yoga Journal,* March 16, 2010, http://www.yogajournal.com/article/philosophy/love-in-full-bloom/.

56 Gundrun Rudolfsson and Ingela Berggren, "Nursing Students' Perspectives on the Patient and the Impact of the Nursing Culture: A Meta-synthesis," *Journal of Nursing Management* 20, no. 6 (2012): 771-81, doi:10.1111/j.1365-2834.2012.01470.x.

57 Thich Nhat Hanh, *The Mindfulness Survival Kit: Five Essential Practices* (Berkeley, CA: Parallax Press, 2014).

58 National Research Council, *To Err is Human: Building a Safer Health System* (Washington, DC: The National Academies Press, 2000).

59 Ross McL. Wilson et al., "The Quality in Australian Health Care Study," *Medical Journal of Australia,* 163 (1995):458-71.

60 UK Department of Health, *An Organisation with a Memory* (London: The Stationery Office, 2000).

61 Tom Muha, "Medical Errors: Why Don't Nurses Speak Up?" *NurseTogether.com* June 26, 2014, http://www.nursetogether.com/medical-errors-why-people-who-see-somethin.

62 Eileen Relihan et al., "The Impact of a Set of Interventions to Reduce Interruptions and Distractions to Nurses during Medication Administration," *Quality & Safety in Health Care* 19, no. 52 (2010): 1-6, doi:10.1136/qshc.2009.036871.

63   Johanna I. Westbrook et al., "Association of Interruptions with an Increased Risk and Severity of Medication Administration Errors," *Archives of Internal Medicine* 170 (2010): 683-90.

64   Juliana J. Brixey et al., "The Roles of MDs and RNs as Initiators and Recipients of Interruptions in Workflow," *International Journal of Medical Informatics* 79, no. 6 (2010): 109-15. doi:10.1016/j.ijmedinf.2008.08.007.

65   Linda McGillis Hall et al., "Going Blank: Factors Contributing to Interruptions to Nurses' Work and Related Outcomes," *Journal of Nursing Management* 18, no. 8 (2010): 1040-47, doi:10.1111/j.1365-2834.2010.01166.x.

66   Nursingprocess.com, "Nursing Process Steps," http://www.nursingprocess.org/Nursing-Process-Steps.html.

67   Tanja Manser and Simon Foster, "Effective Handover Communication: An Overview of Research and Improvement Efforts," *Clinical Anaesthesiology* 25, no. 2 (2011): 181-91, doi:10.1016/j.bpa.2011.02.006.

68   Darrell J. Solet et al., "Lost in Translation: Challenges and Opportunities in Physician-to-Physician Communication during Patient Handovers," *Academic Medicine* 80, no. 12 (2005): 1094-99.

69   Joint Commission International, "About JCI," http://www.jointcommissioninternational.org/about/.

70   Deborah Tregunno, "Transferring Clients Safely: Know your Client and Know your Team," *College of Nurses of Ontario Project Report: Transfer of Accountability Knowledge Translation* April 29, 2009, http://www.cno.org/Global/docs/policy/TransferringClientsSafelyApril2009.pdf, p. 1.

71   Steve Boorman, *NHS Health & Well-Being Improvement Framework* (London: Crown, 2009).

72   Patricia Reid Ponte and Paula Koppel, "Cultivating Mindfulness to Enhance Nursing Practice," *American Journal of Nursing* 115, no. 6 (2015): 48-55, doi:10.1097/01.NAJ.0000466321.46439.17.

73   Jacqueline G. Willingham, "Managing Presenteeism and Disability to Improve Productivity," *Benefits & Compensation Digest* 45, no. 12 (2008): 10-14, http://www.ifebp.org/inforequest/0155525.pdf.

74   University of Massachusetts (UMass) Medical School Center for Mindfulness, "Mobilize your own Inner Resources for Learning, Growing, and Healing," http://www.umassmed.edu/cfm/stress-reduction.

75 Barry Boyce, "The Secret of Success of MBSR," *Mindful*, http://www.mindful.org/in-body-and-mind/mindfulness-based-stress-reduction/the-secret-of-success-for-mbsr.

76 UMass, "Mobilize Your Own Inner Resources."

77 Sheldon Cohen, Tom Kamarck, and Robin Mermelstein, "A Global Measure of Perceived Stress," *Journal of Health and Social Behavior* 24 (1983): 386-96, http://www.jstor.org/stable/2136404.

78 Christina Maslach et al., "Maslach Burnout Inventory (MBI): The Leading Measure of Burnout," *MindGarden.com*, http://www.mindgarden.com/products/mbi.htm.

79 Raes et al., "Construction and Factorial Validation."

80 Wendy Leebov, "The One Skill that Can Transform Health Care," *H&HN: Hospitals & Health Networks* January 21, 2014, http://www.hhnmag.com/display/HHN-news-article.dhtml?dcrPath=/templatedata/HF_Common/NewsArticle/data/HHN/Daily/2014/Jan/012114-article-hospital-patient-experience.

81 Barsade and O'Neill, "What's Love Got to Do with It?"

82 Stanford School of Medicine, "About Compassion Cultivation Training (CCT)," http://ccare.stanford.edu/education/about-compassion-cultivation-training-cct/.

83 Hooria Jazaieri, Kelly McGonigal, Thupten Jinpa, James R. Doty, James J. Gross, and Philippe R. Goldin, "A Randomized Controlled Trial of Compassion Cultivation Training: Effects on Mindfulness, Affect, and Emotion Regulation," *Motivation and Emotion* 38, no. 1 (2013), doi: 10.1007/s11031-013-9368-z

84 Hooria Jazaieri, et al., "Enhancing compassion: A randomized controlled trial of a Compassion Cultivation Training program," *Journal of Happiness Studies* 14, no. 4 (2013): 1113-1126, doi: 10.1007/s10902-012-9373-z.

85 Hooria Jazaieri, et al., "A wandering mind is a less caring mind: Daily experience sampling during Compassion Meditation Training," *The Journal of Positive Psychology* 11, no. 1 (2015), doi: 10.1080/17439760.2015.1025418.

86 Point of Care Foundation, "Schwartz Centre Rounds: Frequently Asked Questions," http://www.pointofcarefoundation.org.uk/Downloads/Schwartz-Center-Rounds-FAQs.pdf.

[87] Julie Rosen and Thomas Lynch Jr., "The Talking Cure: Schwartz Center Rounds Foster Compassion and Collaboration," *Journal of Cancer Education* 23, no. 3 (2008): 195-96, doi:10.1080/08858190802244330.

[88] Schwartz Center for Compassionate Healthcare, "Schwartz Center Rounds," http://www.theschwartzcenter.org/supporting-caregivers/schwartz-center-rounds/.

[89] Beth A. Lown and Colleen F. Manning, "The Schwartz Center Rounds: Evaluation of an Interdisciplinary Approach to Enhancing Patient-Centered Communication, Teamwork, and Provider Support," *Academic Medicine* 85, no. 6 (2010): 1073-81, doi:10.1097/ACM.0b013e3181dbf741.

[90] Ibid.

[91] Joanna Goodrich, "Supporting Hospital Staff to Provide Compassionate Care: Do Schwartz Center Rounds Work in English Hospitals?" *Journal of the Royal Society of Medicine* 105 (2012): 117-22, doi:10.1258/jrsm.2011.11018.

References

Allard, Kateri. "How Do I Fail Thee? Let Me Count the Ways." *According to Kateri: A Blog*, December 11, 2013. http://accordingtokateri.com/2013/12/11/how-do-i-fail-thee-let-me-count-the-ways/.

American Psychiatric Association. *Diagnostic and Statistical Manual of Mental Disorders: DSMV*. 5th ed. Arlington, VA: Author, 2013.

Anderson, Amanda. "The Poetry of the IV." *This Nurse Wonders*, September 16, 2014. http://thisnursewonders.com/2014/09/16/the-poetry-of-the-iv/.

Anderson, Cherri D., and Ruthie R. Mangino. "Nurse Shift Report: Who Says You Can't Talk in Front of the Patient?" *Nursing Administration Quarterly* 30, no. 2 (2006): 112-22.

Barnard, Laura K., and John F. Curry. "Self-Compassion: Conceptualizations, Correlates, & Interventions." *Review of General Psychology* 15, no. 4 (2011): 289–303.

Barsade, Sigal G., and Olivia A. O'Neill. "What's Love Got to Do with It? A Longitudinal Study of the Culture of Companionate Love and Employee and Client Outcomes in a Long-term Care Setting." *Administrative Science Quarterly* 59, no. 4 (2014): 551-98. doi:10.1177/0001839214538636.

Beach, Mary Catherine, Debra Roter, P. Todd Korthuis, Ronald M. Epstein, Victoria Sharp, Neda Ratanawongsa, Jonathan Cohn et al. "A Multicenter Study of Physician Mindfulness and Health Care Quality." *Annals of Family Medicine* 11, no. 5 (2013): 421-28. doi:10.1370/afm.1507.

Beddoe, Amy E., and Susan O. Murphy. "Does Mindfulness Decrease Stress and Foster Empathy among Nursing students?" *Journal of Nursing Education* 43, no. 7 (2004): 305-12.

Benson, Herbert. *The Relaxation Response*. New York: William Morrow, 1975.

Bishop, Anne H., and John R. Scudder Jr. *The Practical, Moral, and Personal Sense of Nursing: A Phenomenological Philosophy of Practice*. Albany: State University of New York Press, 1990.

Boccio, Frank Jude. "Love in Full Bloom." *Yoga Journal*, March 16, 2010. http://www.yogajournal.com/article/philosophy/love-in-full-bloom/.

Boorman, Steve. *NHS Health & Well-Being Improvement Framework*. London: Crown, 2009.

Boorstein, Sylvia. *Don't Just Do Something, Sit There: A Mindfulness Retreat with Sylvia Boorstein*. San Francisco: Harper One, 1996.

Boyce, Barry. "The Secret of Success of MBSR." *Mindful*. http://www.mindful.org/in-body-and-mind/mindfulness-based-stress-reduction/the-secret-of-success-for-mbsr.

Boyle, Deborah A. "Countering Compassion Fatigue: A Requisite Nursing Agenda." *Online Journal of Issues in Nursing* 16, no. 1 (2011): 1. doi:10.3912/OJIN.Vol16No01Man02.

Brault, Robert. *Round Up the Usual Subjects: Thoughts on Just About Everything*. Createspace Independent Publishing, 2014.

Brixey, Juliana J., David J. Robinson, James P. Turley, and Jiajie Zhang. "The Roles of MDs and RNs as Initiators and Recipients of Interruptions in Workflow." *International Journal of Medical Informatics* 79, no. 6 (2010): 109-15. doi:10.1016/j.ijmedinf.2008.08.007.

Brown, Kirk Warren, and Richard M. Ryan. "The Benefits of Being Present: Mindfulness and its Role in Psychological Well-Being." *Journal of Personality and Social Psychology* 84, no. 4 (2003): 822-48, doi:10.1037/0022-3514.84.4.822.

Bush, Nancy Jo, and Deborah A. Boyle. *Self-healing through Reflection: A Workbook for Nurses*. Pittsburgh, PA: Hygeia Media, 2001.

Carlson, Linda E., and Michael Speca. *Mindfulness-Based Cancer Recovery*. Oakland, CA: New Harbringer Publications, 2010.

Carson, James W., Francis J. Keefe, Thomas R. Lynch, Kimberly M. Carson, Veerainder Goli, Anne Marie Fras, and Steven R. Thorp. "Loving-Kindness Meditation for Chronic Low Back Pain: Results from a Pilot Trial." *Journal of Holistic Nursing* 23, no. 3 (2005): 287-304. doi:10.1177/0898010105277651.

Chapman, Susan Gillis. *The Five Keys to Mindful Communication: Using Deep Listening and Mindful Speech to Strengthen Relationships, Heal Conflicts, and Accomplish Your Goals*. Boston: Shambhala, 2012.

Chödrön, Pema. *Start Where You Are: A Guide to Compassionate Living*. Boston: Shambhala Publications, 2001.

Chödrön, Pema. *The Wisdom of No Escape and the Path of Loving-Kindness*. Boston: Shambhala Publications, 2010.

Clark, Robin Craig. *The Garden: A Tranquil Ode to Love*. Melbourne, AU: Peliguin Publishing, 2005.

CMF-USA. "Compassion-Focused Therapy." http://www.compassionfocusedtherapy.com/.

Cohen, Marlene Z., Katherine Brown-Saltzman, and Marilyn J. Shirk. "Taking Time for Support." *Oncology Nursing Forum* 28 (2004): 25-27.

Cohen, Sheldon, Tom Kamarck, and Robin Mermelstein. "A Global Measure of Perceived Stress." *Journal of Health and Social Behavior* 24 (1983): 386-96. http://www.jstor.org/stable/2136404.

Cohen-Katz, Joanne, Susan D. Wiley, Terry Capuano, Debra M. Baker, and Shauna Shapiro. "The Effects of Mindfulness-Based Stress Reduction on Nurse Stress and Burnout, Part II: A Quantitative and Qualitative Study." *Holistic Nursing Practice*, 19, no. 1 (2005): 26-35.

Compassionate Mind Foundation. "Welcome to the Compassionate Mind Foundation." *Compassionatemind.org.* http://www.compassionatemind.co.uk/.

Condon, Paul, and David DeSteno. "Compassion for One Reduces Punishment for Another." *Journal of Experimental Social Psychology* 47 (2011): 698-701. doi:10.1016/j.jesp.2010.11.016.

Condon, Paul, Gaëlle Desbordes, Willa B. Miller, and David DeSteno. "Meditation Increases Compassionate Responses to Suffering." *Psychological Science* 24, no. 10 (2013). doi: 10.1177/0956797613485603.

Dalai Lama, and Howard C. Cutler. *The Art of Happiness: A Handbook for Living.* 10th anniv. ed. London: Hodder Paperbacks, 2009.

Dent, Sean."5 Tips for a Great Hand-Off Report," November 23, 2012. http://scrubsmag.com/giving-a-good-report/

Dignity Health. "Scientific Literature Review Shows Health Care Delivered with Kindness and Compassion Leads to Faster Healing, Reduced Pain," press release, November 12, 2014. http://www.reuters.com/article/2014/11/12/ca-dignity-health-idUSnBw125352a+100+BSW20141112.

Dines, Christopher. *Mindfulness Meditation: Bringing Mindfulness into Everyday Life.* London: La Petite Fleur Publishing, 2014.

Diomidous, Marianna, Zoe Mpizopoulou, Athena Kalokairinou, I. Mprokalaki, Dimitrios Zikos, and Theophanis Katostaras. "Descriptive Study of Nursing Students' Motives to Choose Nursing as a Career." *Greek Journal of Nursing Science* 2, no. 5: (2013), 60-63.

Di Pellegrino,Giuseppe, Luciano Fadiga, Leonardo Fogassi, Vittorio Gallese, and Giacomo Rizzolatti. "Understanding Motor Events: A Neurophysiological Study," *Experimental Brain Research* 91, no. 1 (1992), 176-180.

Domrose, Cathryn. "Meditation Offers Benefits for Nurses and Patients." *Nurse.com*. June 6, 2010. http://news.nurse.com/article/20100606/NATIONAL02/306060011/-1/frontpage

Epstein, Ronald M. "Mindful Practice." *Journal of the American Medical Association* 282, no. 9 (1999): 833-39.

Frankl, Viktor. *Man's Search for Meaning: An Introduction to Logotherapy*. Boston: Beacon Press, 1959.

Frisvold, Melissa H., Ruth Lindquist, and Cynthia Pedan McAlpine. "Living Life in the Balance at Midlife: Lessons Learned from Mindfulness." *Western Journal of Nursing Research* 34, no. 2 (2012): 265-78.

Germer, Christopher. "Mindful Self-Compassion Training." *Mindful Self-Compassion*. http://www.mindfulselfcompassion.org/mscprogram.php.

Germer, Christopher K. *The Mindful Path to Self-Compassion: Freeing Yourself from Destructive Thoughts and Emotions*. New York: Guilford Press, 2009.

Gilbert, Paul, and Choden. *Mindful Compassion*. London: Constable Robinson, 2013.

Ginsberg, Alan. "Negative Capability: Kerouac's Buddhist Ethic." In *Everyday Mind*, edited by Jean Smith, 96. New York: Riverhead Books, 1977.

Goldstein, Joseph. *Insight Meditation: The Practice of Freedom*. Boston: Shambhala Publications, 1993.

Gomez, Marc. "Can Mindfulness Prevent Potentially Hazardous Errors?" *Safety.BLR*, January 17, 2014. http://safety.blr.com/workplace-safety-news/safety-administration/safety-general/Can-mindfulness-prevent-potentially-hazardous-erro/

Goodrich, Joanna. "Supporting Hospital Staff to Provide Compassionate Care: Do Schwartz Center Rounds Work in English Hospitals?" *Journal of the Royal Society of Medicine* 105 (2012): 117-22. doi:10.1258/jrsm.2011.11018.

Gray-Toft, Pamela, and James G. Anderson. "The Nursing Stress Scale: Development of an Instrument." *Journal of Behavioral Assessment* 3, no. 1 (1981): 11-23. doi:10.1007/BF01321348.

Greater Good. "Quizzes." http://greatergood.berkeley.edu/quizzes/take_quiz/1.

Hafenbrack, Andrew, Zoe Kinias, and Sigal Barsade. "Debiasing the Mind through Meditation: Mindfulness and the Sunk-Cost Bias." *Psychological Science*25, no. 2 (2013) 369-76.

Halifax, Joan. "Compassion and the True Meaning of Empathy." Filmed December 2010. TED video, 14:01. Posted September 2011. https://www.ted.com/talks/joan_halifax/transcript?language=en.

———. "G.R.A.C.E. for Nurses: Cultivating Compassion in Nurse/Patient Interactions." *Journal of Nursing Education and Practice* 4, no. 1 (2014): 121-28.

Hall, Linda McGillis, Mary Ferguson-Paré, Elizabeth Peter, Debbie White, Jeanne Besner, Anne Chisholm, Ella Ferris et al. "Going Blank: Factors Contributing to Interruptions to Nurses' Work and Related Outcomes." *Journal of Nursing Management* 18, no. 8 (2010): 1040-47. doi:10.1111/j.1365-2834.2010.01166.x.

Halligan, Aidan. "The NHS Needs Compassionate Leadership." *Journal of Holistic Healthcare* 11, no. 1 (2014): 4.

Hare, Julius Charles, and Augustus William Hare. *Guesses at Truth: by Two Brothers*. London: John Taylor, 1827. http://www.archive.org/stream/guessesattruthby00hareiala/guessesattruthby00hareiala_djvu.txt

Hendrich, Ann, Marilyn P. Chow, Boguslaw A. Skierczynski, and Zhenqiang Lu. "A 36-Hospital Time and Motion Study: How do Medical-Surgical Nurses Spend their Time?" *The Permanente Journal* 12, no. 3 (2008): 25-34.

Herrmann, Dorothy. *Helen Keller: A Life.* Chicago: University of Chicago Press, 1999.

Hoge, Elizabeth A., Maxine M. Chen, Esther Orr, Christina A. Metcalf, Laura E. Fischer, Mark H. Pollock, Immaculata DeVivo et al. "Loving-Kindness Meditation Practice Associated with Longer Telomeres in Women." *Brain Behavior and Immunity* 32 (2013): 159-63. doi:10.1016/j.bbi.2013.04.005.

Hölzel, Britta K., James Carmody, Mark Vangel, Christina Congleton, Sita M. Yerramsetti, Tim Gard, Sara W. Lazar. "Mindfulness Practice Leads to Increases in Regional Brain Gray Matter Density." *Psychiatry Research: Neuroimaging* 191, no. 1(2011): 36.doi:10.1016/j.pscychresns.2010.08.006.

Holzman, David C. "What's in a Color? The Unique Human Health Effects of Blue Light." *Environmental Health Perspectives* 118, no. 1 (2010): A22-A27. doi:10.1289/ehp.118-a22.

Janakabhivamsa, Chanmyay Sayadaw U. "Lectures on Insight Meditation (1992)." *Vipassana Meditation.* Last modified October 23, 2014. http://www.myanmarnet.net/nibbana/chanmyay.htm.

Jazaieri, Hooria, Kelly McGonigal, Thupten Jinpa, James R. Doty, James J. Gross, and Philippe R. Goldin." A Randomized Controlled Trial of Compassion Cultivation Training: Effects on Mindfulness, Affect, and Emotion Regulation," *Motivation and Emotion* 38, no. 1 (2013). doi: 10.1007/s11031-013-9368-z.

Jazaieri, Hooria, Geshe Thupten Jinpa, Kelly McGonigal, Erika L. Rosenberg, Joel Finkelstein, Emiliana Simon-Thomas, Margaret Cullen, James R. Doty, James J. Gross, and Philippe R. Goldin. "Enhancing Compassion: A Randomized Controlled Trial of a Compassion Cultivation Training program," *Journal of Happiness Studies* 14, no. 4 (2013): 1113-1126. doi: 10.1007/s10902-012-9373-z.

Jazaieri, Hooria, Ihno A. Lee, Kelly McGonigal, Thupten Jinpa, James R. Doty, James J. Gross, and Philippe R. Goldin. "A Wandering Mind is a Less Caring Mind: Daily Experience Sampling During Compassion Meditation Training." *The Journal of Positive Psychology* 11, no. 1 (2015). doi: 10.1080/17439760.2015.1025418.

Joinson, Clara. "Coping with Compassion Fatigue." *Nursing* 22 (1992): 116-21.

Joint Commission International. "About JCI." http://www.jointcommissioninternational.org/about/

June, Kyung Ja, and Sung-Hyu Cho. "Low-Back Pain and Work-Related Factors Using Nurses in Intensive Care Units." *Journal of Clinical Nursing* 20, no. 3-4 (2011): 479-87. doi:10.1111/j.1365-2702.2010.03210.x.

Kabat-Zinn, Jon. *Coming to our Senses: Healing Ourselves and the World through Mindfulness.* New York: Hyperion, 2005.

———. *Full Catastrophe Living: Using the Wisdom of your Body and Mind to Face Stress, Pain, and Illness.* New York: Dell Publishing, 1991.

———. *Letting Everything Become Your Teacher: 100 Lessons in Mindfulness.* New York: Delta, 2009.

———. "Mindful Yoga, Movement and Meditation." *Yoga Chicago Magazine,* March/April2005. http://yogachicago.com/2014/03/mindful-yoga-movement-and-meditation/.

———. *Wherever You Go, There You Are: Mindfulness Meditation in Everyday Life.* New York: Hyperion, 1994.

Kay, Kate, and Nel Glass. "Debunking the Manual Handling Myth: An Investigation of Manual Handling Knowledge and Practices in the Australian Private Health Sector." *International Journal of Nursing Practice* 17 (2011): 231-237. doi:10.1111/j.1440-172x.2011.01930.x.

Keltner, Dacher. "We Are Built to Be Kind." *Fig. 1, University of California*, YouTube video, 4:36. Posted December 2, 2014. https://www.youtube.com/watch?v=SsWs6bf7tvI.

Killingsworth, Matthew A. and Daniel T. Gilbert. "A Wandering Mind Is an Unhappy Mind." *Science* 330, no. 6006 (2010): 932. doi: 10.1126/science.1192439.

Koerner, Joellen Goertz. *Healing Presence: The Essence of Nursing*. New York: Springer Publishing, 2011.

Kok, Bethany E., Kimberly A. Coffey, Michael A. Cohn, Lahnna I. Catalino, Tanya Vacharkulksemsuk, Sara B. Algoe, Mary Brantley et al. "How Positive Emotions Build Physical Health: Perceived Positive Social Connections Account for the Upward Spiral between Positive Emotions and Vagal Tone." *Psychological Science* 24, no. 7 (2013): 1123-32. doi:10.1177/0956797612470827.

Kongtrul, Jamgon. *The Torch of Certainty*. Translated by Judith Hanson. Boston: Shambhala Publications, 2010.

Kornfield, Jack. *Buddha's Little Instruction Book*. London: Rider Books, 1996.

——— *The Wise Heart: A Guide to the Universal Teachings of Buddhist Psychology*. New York: Random House, 2008.

Krasner, Michael S., Ronald M. Epstein, Howard Beckman, Anthony L. Suchman, Benjamin Chapman, Christopher J. Mooney, and Timothy E. Quill. "Association of an Educational Program in Mindful Communication with Burnout, Empathy, and Attitudes among Primary Care Physicians." *Journal of the American Medical Association* 302, no. 12 (2009):1284-93. doi:0.1001/jama.2009.1384.

Kriseman, Nancy L. *The Mindful Caregiver: Finding Ease in the Caregiver Journey*. Lanham, MD: Rowman & Littlefield, 2014.

Krishnamurti, Jiddu. *The First and Last Freedom.* Brandean, UK: Krishnamurti Foundation Trust, 1954.

L'Amour, Louis. *Bendigo Shafter.* New York: Bantam Books,1979.

Lane, Christie. "Yoga and Mindfulness: Perspective of an RN Yoga Instructor." *Journal of Nursing, UC San Diego* (Summer 2014): 7-9. https://health.ucsd.edu/medinfo/nursing/Documents/Nursing-Sum-2014.pdf.

Lao-tzu. *Tao Te Ching.* Edited by Stephen Mitchell. New York: Harper Perennial, 1992.

Leebov, Wendy. "The One Skill that Can Transform Health Care." *H&HN: Hospitals & Health Networks,* January 21, 2014. http://www.hhnmag.com/display/HHN-news-article.dhtml?dcrPath=/templatedata/HF_Common/NewsArticle/data/HHN/Daily/2014/Jan/012114-article-hospital-patient-experience.

Levine, Stephen. *A Year to Live: How to Live This Year as if It Were Your Last.* New York: Bell Tower, 1997.

Lokos, Allan. *Pocket Peace: Effective Practices for Enlightened Living.* New York: Jeremy P. Tarcher/Penguin, 2010.

Lombardo, Barbara, and Caryl Eyre. «Compassion Fatigue: A Nurse's Primer.» *Online Journal of Issues in Nursing*16, no. 1 (2011): 3. doi:10.3912/OJIN.Vol16No01Man03.

Lown, Beth A., and Colleen F. Manning. "The Schwartz Center Rounds: Evaluation of an Interdisciplinary Approach to Enhancing Patient-Centered Communication, Teamwork, and Provider Support." *Academic Medicine* 85, no. 6 (2010): 1073-81. doi:10.1097/ACM.0b013e3181dbf741.

Manser, Tanja, and Simon Foster. "Effective Handover Communication: An Overview of Research and Improvement Efforts." *Clinical Anaesthesiology* 25, no. 2 (2011): 181–91. doi:10.1016/j.bpa.2011.02.006.

Maslach, Christina, Susan E. Jackson, Michael P. Leiter, Wilmar B. Schaufeli, and Richard L. Schwab. "Maslach Burnout Inventory (MBI): The Leading Measure of Burnout." *MindGarden.com.* http://www.mindgarden.com/products/mbi.htm.

Mate, Gabor. *In the Realm of Hungry Ghosts: Close Encounters with Addiction.* Berkeley,CA:North Atlantic Books, 2010.

Mathieu, Françoise. "Compassion Fatigue." In *Encyclopedia of Trauma: An Interdisciplinary Guide*, edited by Charles R. Figley, 136-39. Los Angeles: SAGE, 2012.

Maytum, Jennifer, Mary Heiman, and Ann Garwick. "Compassion Fatigue and Burnout in Nurses Who Work with Children with Chronic Conditions and Their Families." *Journal of Pediatric Healthcare* 18, no. 4 (2004): 171-179.

Melvin, Christina S. "Professional Compassion Fatigue: What is the True Cost of Nurses Caring for the Dying?" *International Journal of Palliative Nursing* 18, no. 12 (2012): 606-611.

Meredith, Nancy. "Use the 'Ring of Theory' as a Guide to Avoid Common Mistakes when Talking to Mesothelioma Patients and their Family." *MesotheliomaHelp.org* (blog). http://www.mesotheliomahelp.org/2013/09/use-the-ring-of-theory-as-a-guide-to-avoid-communication-mistakes-when-talking-to-mesothelioma-patients-and-their-family/.

Miller, Lyle H., Alma Dell Smith, and Larry Rothstein. *The Stress Solution: An Action Plan to Manage the Stress in Your Life.* Edited by Larry Rothstein. New York: Pocket Books, 1994.

Muha, Tom. "Medical Errors: Why Don't Nurses Speak Up?" *NurseTogether.com,* June 26, 2014. http://www.nursetogether.com/medical-errors-why-people-who-see-somethin.

National Research Council. *To Err is Human: Building a Safer Health System.* Washington, DC: National Academies Press, 2000.

Neff, Kristin D. "The Development and Validation of a Scale to Measure Self-Compassion." *Self and Identity* 2 (2003): 223-50. doi:10.1080/15298860309027.

Neff, Kristin D., and Christopher K. Germer. "A Pilot Study and Randomized Controlled Trial of the Mindful Self-Compassion Program." *Journal of Clinical Psychology* 69 (2013): 28-44.

Neu, Diann. "Blessing Our Hands," adapted by Corlette Pierson from "In Praise of Hands." *Waterwheel* Winter (1989).

Neufeld, Kenley. "I Love Technology: Practicing Mindfulness and Valuing Technology." *Mindfulness and Meditation*, March 30, 2014. https://medium.com/mindfulness-and-meditation/i-love-technology-364cc2272918.

Newton, John. *The Amazing Works of John Newton*. Edited by Harold J. Chadwick. Alachua, FL: Bridge-Logos, 2009.

Nhat Hanh, Thich. *Be Free Where You Are*. Berkeley, CA: Parallax Press, 2002.

———. *Fear: Essential Wisdom for Getting through the Storm*. New York: Harper Collins, 2012.

———. *For a Future to Be Possible: Buddhist Ethics for Everyday Life*. Berkeley, CA: Parallax Press, 1993.

———. *Living Buddha, Living Christ*. New York: Riverhead Books,1995.

———. *The Long Road Turns to Joy: A Guide to Walking Meditation*. Berkeley, CA: Parallax Press, 2006.

———. *The Mindfulness Survival Kit: Five Essential Practices*. Berkeley, CA: Parallax Press, 2014.

———. *The Miracle of Mindfulness: An Introduction to the Practice of Meditation*. Boston: Beacon Press, 1999.

———. "Oprah Winfrey Talks with Thich Nhat Hahn Excerpt: Powerful." YouTube video. Posted May 2013. https://www.youtube.com/watch?v=NJ9UtuWfs3U.

————. *The Path of Emancipation: Talks from a 21-Day Mindfulness Retreat.* Berkeley, CA: Parallax Press, 2000.

————. *Work: How to Find Joy and Meaning in Each Hour of the Day.* Berkeley, CA: Parallax Press, 2012.

Nhat Hanh, Thich, and Lilian Cheung. *Savor: Mindful Eating, Mindful Life.* New York: Harper Collins, 2010.

Nursingprocess.com. "Nursing Process Steps." http://www.nursingprocess.org/Nursing-Process-Steps.html.

O'Donohue, John. *To Bless the Space Between Us: A Book of Blessings.* USA: Doubleday, 2008.

Palmer, Parker J. *Let Your Life Speak: Listening for the Voice of Vocation.* Hoboken, NJ: John Wiley & Sons, 2000.

Patch Adams. Directed by Tom Shadyac. Hollywood, CA: Universal Studios, 1998.

Pezzolesi, Cinzia, Maisoon Ghaleb, Andrzej Kostrzewski, and Soraya Dhillon. "Is Mindful Reflective Practice the Way Forward to Reduce Medication Errors?" *International Journal of Pharmacy Practice* 21, no. 6 (2013): 413-16. doi:10.1111/ijpp.12031.

Point of Care Foundation. "Schwartz Centre Rounds: Frequently Asked Questions." http://www.pointofcarefoundation.org.uk/Downloads/Schwartz-Center-Rounds-FAQs.pdf.

Ponte, Patricia Reid, and Paula Koppel. "Cultivating Mindfulness to Enhance Nursing Practice." *American Journal of Nursing* 115, no. 6 (2015): 48-55. doi:10.1097/01.NAJ.0000466321.46439.17.

Puddicombe, Andy. "The Mindful Use of Technology." *Psychology Today,* July 9,2013. https://www.psychologytoday.com/blog/get-some-headspace/201307/the-mindful-use-technology

Raab, Kelley. "Mindfulness, Self-Compassion, and Empathy among Health Care Professionals: A Review of the Literature." *Journal of Health Care Chaplaincy* 20, no. 3 (2014): 95-108.doi:10.1080/0 8854726.2014.913876.

Radcliffe, Mark. "Compassion Is No Harder to Measure than Rain." *Nursing Times* 106, no. 17 (2010): 23.

Raes, Filip, Elizabeth Pommier, Kristin D. Neff, and Dinska Van Gucht. "Construction and Factorial Validation of a Short Form of the Self-compassion Scale." *Clinical Psychology & Psychotherapy* 18 (2011): 250-55. doi:0.1002/cpp.702.

Ravindra, Ravi. *The Wisdom of Patanjali's Yoga Sutras: A New Translation and Guide.* Sandpoint, ID: Morning Light Press, 2009.

Relihan, Eileen, Valerie O'Brien, Sharon O'Hara, and Bernard Silke. "The Impact of a Set of Interventions to Reduce Interruptions and Distractions to Nurses during Medication Administration." *Quality & Safety in Health Care* [now BMJ Quality & Safety] 19, no. 52 (2010): 1-6. doi:10.1136/qshc.2009.036871.

Remen, Rachel Naomi. *Kitchen Table Wisdom: Stories that Heal.* New York: Riverhead Books, 1996.

Ricard, Matthieu. "Empathy Fatigue-2." Posted October 9, 2013. http://www.matthieuricard.org/en/blog/posts/empathy-fatigue-2

Rilke, Rainer Maria. Selected Letters of Rainer Maria Rilke, 1902-1926. London: Macmillan, 1947.

Rosen, Julie, and Thomas Lynch Jr. "The Talking Cure: Schwartz Center Rounds Foster Compassion and Collaboration." *Journal of Cancer Education* 23, no. 3 (2008): 195-96. doi:10.1080/08858190802244330.

Royal College of Nursing. *Good Practice for Handling Feedback.* London: Royal College of Nursing, 2014.

Rudolfsson, Gundrun, and Ingela Berggren. "Nursing Students' Perspectives on the Patient and the Impact of the Nursing Culture: A Meta-synthesis." *Journal of Nursing Management* 20, no. 6 (2012): 771-81. doi:10.1111/j.1365-2834.2012.01470.x.

Rumi. "The Sunrise Ruby." In *The Essential Rumi*, translated by Coleman Barks, 100. San Francisco: Harper Collins, 1995.

Salzberg, Sharon. *Loving-Kindness: The Revolutionary Art of Happiness.* Boston: Shambhala Publications, 2002.

——. *Real Happiness at Work: Meditations for Accomplishment, Achievement, and Peace.* New York: Workman Publishing Company, 2013.

——. *Real Happiness: The Power of Meditation: A 28-Day Program.* New York: Workman, 2010.

Schwartz Center for Compassionate Healthcare. "Schwartz Center Rounds." http://www.theschwartzcenter.org/supporting-caregivers/schwartz-center-rounds/.

Seppala, Emma M., Cendri A. Hutcherson, Dong T. H. Nguyen, James K. Doty, and James J. Gross. "Loving-Kindness Meditation: A Tool to Improve Healthcare Provider Compassion, Resilience, and Patient Care." *Journal of Compassionate Healthcare* 1 (2014): 5. doi:10.1186/s40639-014-0005-9.

Shapira, Leah B., and Myriam Mongrain. "The Benefits of Self-Compassion and Optimism Exercises for Individuals Vulnerable to Depression." *Journal of Positive Psychology* 5 (2010): 377-89.

Shapiro, Shauna, and Linda Carlson. *The Art and Science of Mindfulness: Integrating Mindfulness into Psychology and the Helping Professions.* Washington, DC: American Psychological Society, 2009.

Shuman, Jill. "Enhancing Patient Adherence: And What to Do When All Else Fails." *Primary Care Network*, October 19, 2010. http://www.primaryissues.org/2010/10/enhancing-patient-adherence-and-what-to-do-when-all-else-fails/.

Silk, Susan, and Barry Goldman. "How Not to Say the Wrong Thing." *Los Angeles Times*, April 7, 2013. http://articles.latimes.com/2013/apr/07/opinion/la-oe-0407-silk-ring-theory-20130407.

Solet, Darrell J., Michael J. Norvell, Gale H. Rutan, and Richard M. Frankel. "Lost in Translation: Challenges and Opportunities in Physician-to-Physician Communication during Patient Handovers." *Academic Medicine* 80, no. 12 (2005): 1094-99.

Stamm, B. Hudnall. "Professional Quality of Life: Compassion Satisfaction and Fatigue (ProQOL)." Version 5. Last modified 2009. http://www.proqol.org.

Stanford University Center for Compassion and Altruism Research and Education. "About Compassion Cultivation Training." http://ccare.stanford.edu/education/about-compassion-cultivation-training-cct/.

Suttie, Jill. "How to Increase Compassion at Work." *Greater Good*, February 16, 2015. http://greatergood.berkeley.edu/article/item/how_to_increase_compassion_at_work.

Thera, Nyanaponika. "The Four Sublime States: Contemplations on Love, Compassion, Sympathetic Joy, and Equanimity." *Access to Insight (Legacy Edition)*, November 30, 2013. http://www.accesstoinsight.org/lib/authors/nyanaponika/wheel006.html.

Tilbrook, Helen E., Helen Cox, Catherine E. Hewitt, Arthur Ricky Kang'ombe, Ling-Hsiang Chuang, Salmini Jayakody, John D. Alpin et al. "Yoga for Chronic Low-Back Pain: A Randomized Trial." *Annals of Intern Medicine* 155 (2011): 569-78. doi:10.7326/0003-4819-155-9-201111010-00003.

Tolle, Eckhart. *A New Earth: Awakening to Your Life's Purpose*. New York: Penguin, 2008.

———. *The Power of Now: A Guide to Spiritual Enlightenment*. Novato, CA: New World Library, 1999.

Tonelli, Makenzie E., and Amy B. Wachholtz. "Meditation-Based, Treatment-Yielding, Immediate Relief for Meditation Naïve Migraineurs." *Pain Management Nursing* 15, no. 1 (2014): 36-40. doi:10.1016/j.pmn.2012.04.002.

Tregunno, Deborah. "Transferring Clients Safely: Know Your Client and Know Your Team." *College of Nurses of Ontario Project Report: Transfer of Accountability Knowledge Translation*, April 29, 2009. http://www.cno.org/Global/docs/policy/TransferringClientsSafelyApril2009.pdf.

UK Department of Health. *An Organisation with a Memory*. London: The Stationery Office, 2000.

University of Massachusetts (UMass) Medical School Center for Mindfulness. "Mobilize Your Own Inner Resources for Learning, Growing, and Healing." http://www.umassmed.edu/cfm/stress-reduction/.

University of Wisconsin Department of Family Medicine and Community Health. "1. Pause (Practice In Your Practice)." http://www.fammed.wisc.edu/mindfulness/pip-pause/.

US Department of Labor, Bureau of Labor Statistics. "Injuries, Illnesses, and Fatalities." Last modified June 19, 2015. http://www.bls.gov/iif/oshfaq1.htm#q16.

Wallis, Sharyn. "Nursing Handover Research Project: How is Nursing Handover Talked about in the Literature?" Master's thesis, Waikato Institute of Technology, Hamilton, New Zealand, 2010. http://researcharchive.wintec.ac.nz/964/.

Ward, Jennifer. "The Importance of Teamwork in Nursing." *nursetogether.com*, January 14, 2013. http://www.nursetogether.com/the-importance-of-teamwork-in-nursing.

Weng, Helen Y., Andrew S. Fox, Alexander J. Shackman, Diane E. Stodola, Jessica Z. K. Caldwell, Matthew C. Olson, Gregory M. Rogers et al. "Compassion Training Alters Altruism and Neural Responses to Suffering." *Psychological Science 24* (2013): 1171-80. doi:1177/0956797612469537.

Westbrook, Johanna I., Amanda Woods, Marilyn I. Rob, William T. M. Dunsmuir, and Richard O. Day. "Association of Interruptions with an Increased Risk and Severity of Medication Administration Errors." *Archives of Internal Medicine* 170 (2010): 683-90.

White, Lacie. "Mindfulness in Nursing: An Evolutionary Concept Analysis." *Journal of Advanced Nursing* 70, no. 2 (2014): 282-94. doi:10.1111/jan.12182.

Wilbur, Mary E. "Leading the Way: Zen at Work; The Use of Meditation in Nursing Practice." *Gastroenterology Nursing* 26, no. 4 (2003): 168-69.

Williams, Mark, John Teasdale, Zindel Segal, and Jon Kabat-Zinn. *The Mindful Way through Depression: Freeing Yourself from Chronic Unhappiness.* New York: Guilford Press, 2007.

Willingham, Jacqueline G. "Managing Presenteeism and Disability to Improve Productivity." *Benefits & Compensation Digest* 45, no. 12 (2008): 10-14. http://www.ifebp.org/inforequest/0155525.pdf.

Wilson, Mary Jane. "A Template for Safe and Concise Handovers." *Medical Surgical Nursing* 16, no. 3 (2007): 201-6. http://www.redorbit.com/news/health/986773/a_template_forsafe_and_concise_handovers/.

Wilson, Ross McL., William B. Runciman, Robert W. Gibberd, Bernadette T. Harrison, Liza Newby, and John D. Hamilton. "The Quality in Australian Health Care Study." *Medical Journal of Australia*, 163 (1995):458-71.

Wolf, Christiane, and Greg Serpa. *A Clinician's Guide to Teaching Mindfulness.* Oakland, CA: New Harbinger Publications, 2015.

Yoder, Elizabeth A. "Caring Too Much: Compassion Fatigue in Nursing." *Applied Nursing Research* 23, no. 4 (2010): 191-197.

Your Guide to Mindfulness-Based Cognitive Therapy. http://mbct.com/.

Zeidan, Fadel, Katherine T. Martucci, Robert A. Kraft, Nakia S. Gordon, John G. McHaffie, and Robert C. Coghill. "Brain Mechanisms Supporting the Modulation of Pain by Mindfulness Meditation." *Journal of Neuroscience* 31, no. 14 (2011): 5540-48.

Index

A

accidents, 132, 134, 181, 295–96

aches, 83, 87, 97, 112, 128, 136–37, 159, 168

activities
anchor, 63, 70
depleting, 92–93

alarms, 114, 116, 304, 306

alpha scale reliability, 330

anger, 61, 90, 106, 108, 120, 122, 154, 181, 190–91, 213–14, 220, 222, 242, 268, 320

animosity, 253, 255

attention, 28–34, 38–40, 42, 48–55, 57–62, 106–8, 110–13, 115–16, 121–24, 238–39, 241, 261–66, 276–78, 282–85, 298–300

attitudes, 19, 66–67, 70, 90, 93, 174, 254–56, 267, 357
mindful, 81–82

autopilot, 31, 45, 47–48, 50–51, 56, 63, 117, 242, 269, 273, 327, 333

Awareness of Emotions in the Body, practice, 121

awareness, 18, 30, 32, 38–39, 83, 110–11, 128–29, 131, 140–41, 159, 161–62, 164–68, 173, 264–66, 318

mindful, 124, 133, 142, 169, 210, 246
open, 264, 266

B

balance, 91–92, 95–97, 102, 118, 159–60, 170, 199, 204, 283, 338, 353

bathroom, 17, 53, 89, 99–100, 102, 130, 168

bladder, 90, 98–99, 103–4

body awareness, 159

body breathing, 83, 265

body language, 184, 261–62

Body Scan, practice, 109

body scan, 18, 38, 108–9, 111–12, 124, 133, 142, 156, 264, 327
short, 112–13, 124, 327

body sensations, 30, 115, 305

breath, mindful, 49, 55, 58, 276, 280, 282–83, 294, 299

breathing, 38–39, 41, 60–61, 63, 83, 110–11, 113, 115, 140–41, 159–62, 166, 168, 224, 227, 239
shallow, 35, 207

breathing space, three-step, 82–86, 156, 296, 327

burnout, 13–14, 18–21, 36, 40, 152, 188–89, 197, 298, 307, 330–31, 336, 346, 351, 357, 359

burnout scale, 330–31

C

caregivers, 17, 77–78, 193, 218–19, 289, 295, 320, 328

CCT (Compassion Cultivation Training), 318–19, 346, 355, 364

challenges, 36, 42–43, 78, 178, 247, 251, 296, 309–10, 314, 317, 319–20, 345, 364

charting, 25–26, 42, 51, 126, 136, 168, 272, 280–82, 295, 297, 303

checklist, 292, 294, 296, 300

chronic low-back pain, 221, 364

code arrest, 79–80, 121

communication, 76, 175, 260, 262, 294–95, 358

compassion
attributes, 179–80, 182
feeling, 176, 191
levels, 200, 213
practices, 13, 18, 37, 192, 197, 215, 224–25, 231, 317–18, 323, 328, 337
practicing, 177, 222

compassionate action, 173, 182, 184

compassionate behaviors, 37, 188, 230

compassion fatigue, 13, 20, 101, 187–89, 191–92, 195–99, 210, 318–19, 329–30, 336, 342–43, 358–59

  antidotes to, 194, 199

  awareness of, 195

Compassion Mantra, practice, 229, 328

computer, 25, 47–48, 54, 84, 100, 113, 146, 281, 297, 299, 302–3, 328

conflict, 43, 147, 217–18, 228, 252–54, 256

contentment, 226–28, 231

coworkers, 43, 46, 99, 177–78, 213–14, 227, 235, 243, 249–50, 254–56, 260, 268, 279, 308, 310

crises, 26, 197, 281, 283

cycle of stress, 152–53, 276

D

distractions, 21, 26, 29, 40, 60, 76, 91, 106, 126, 271–73, 275, 277, 279–83, 285–86, 296

distress, psychological, 220, 222

distressing thoughts, 26, 276

distress tolerance, 180–81

E

eating, 18, 32, 62, 151

  mindful, 61–63, 328, 361

emergencies, 27, 94, 103, 149, 156, 200, 278, 283–84

emotions, 30, 32, 35–36, 120–22, 124, 137, 166–67, 182, 202, 204, 206, 241–42, 264, 266–67, 319

  difficult, 35, 42, 79, 121–24, 161, 191, 197

  painful, 152, 201–2

  positive, 76, 222, 344, 357

empathy, 17, 36, 178, 180–82, 190–92, 198, 216, 319–20, 340, 354, 357, 361

energy, 28, 45, 48, 92, 94, 96, 101, 149, 155, 158–59, 168, 188, 246, 251, 255

errors, 20, 28, 45, 201–2, 243, 272–74, 277–78, 280–82, 285–86, 288, 297, 302, 304, 353

  medication, 58, 272–73, 275, 277, 279

exercise, 74, 92–94, 117, 129, 159, 162, 165, 229

experience

  difficult, 160, 208, 210

  painful, 205

  traumatic, 329

Exploring Difficult Sensations, practice, 137

F

failure, 27, 204–5, 245, 288

families, patient's, 26, 146–47

fatigue, 13, 20, 190, 192, 197, 343, 359, 364

food, 62–63, 94, 236

foot, 61, 95, 97, 110, 119, 287

formal practices, 38, 43, 71, 119, 198, 228, 230–31, 256, 285, 296, 305

Formal Walking Meditation, practice, 118–19, 327

G

goodwill, 215–16, 218, 228, 269

gossip, 251, 254–56

GRACE, practice, 183–86, 328

grief, 122, 192, 195, 197

H

handover report, 287–89, 291–93, 295

hands, 31, 52, 62–65, 104–8, 111, 133, 136, 161, 183, 341, 360

handwashing, mindful, 64, 70, 328

happiness, 16, 76, 119, 215–16, 218–19, 222–23, 226–27, 232, 249, 259, 352, 363

harmony, body experience, 162

healthcare facility, 20, 132, 302, 307, 309, 311, 315, 317–18, 339

healthcare organizations, 81, 321

healthcare workers, 36, 316, 318–19

hostility, 151–52, 225

I

illnesses, 20, 26, 89, 100, 103, 123, 132–33, 143, 249, 262, 268, 335, 341, 356, 365

Informal Walking Meditation, practice, 118

information
important, 176, 291–92, 296
vital, 262, 293–94, 299–300

injuries, 20, 125–26, 128–29, 131–34, 136, 139, 143, 158–59, 162, 169, 334, 341, 365
musculoskeletal, 126, 131

interactions, 30, 38, 40, 49–50, 77, 95, 106, 175, 183–85, 188, 256, 263, 278, 294, 300

interruptions, 27, 76, 273, 279–80, 285, 344–45, 350, 354, 366

IV, 19, 25–27, 36, 42, 68–70, 199, 233, 340, 349

J

judgments, 30, 44, 52, 85, 115, 142, 161, 190, 217, 238, 256, 259, 263, 267–69

L

lift, 125, 128, 131, 134, 164, 166–67, 221

lifting, 83, 119, 125, 127, 131–33, 135, 139, 163

list, to-do, 45, 48, 50, 59, 123, 262

listening, 25, 32, 49, 103, 113, 146, 166, 259, 261, 263, 268, 351, 361
mindful, 114, 262–63, 268–69, 328

love, 13, 17, 29–30, 161, 192, 194, 216, 219, 324, 342, 346, 349, 351, 364

loving-kindness, 37, 192, 215, 217–18, 220–22, 228, 231–32, 269, 319
benefits of, 220, 222
meditation, 18, 216, 220–22, 328, 337, 343, 363
practice, 218–22
program, 221

low-back pain, 341, 356

M

machines, 131, 278, 299, 301–2

MBCT (Mindfulness-Based Cognitive Therapy), 92, 335, 366

MBPM (Mindfulness-Based Pain Management), 335

MBSR (Mindfulness-Based Stress Reduction), 15, 30, 92, 311–15, 321, 335, 346, 350

meals, 18, 46, 62–63, 89–90

medical errors, 271–72, 286–87, 296, 344, 359

medications, 25, 27, 36, 40, 58, 168, 173, 271–72, 275, 277, 279, 284, 292, 294, 297–98

administering, 27, 274, 279

meditation, 41–42, 75, 118–19, 124, 156–59, 198, 225, 229, 334, 336–37, 340, 342–43, 352–56, 360, 363

Mindful Attention Awareness Scale, 31, 77, 313

Mindful Balance, practice, 95, 327

Mindful Breathing, practice, 39

Mindful Check-in, practice, 105

Mindful Foot Care, practice, 98

Mindful Hands, practice, 107

mindful
communication, 259–61, 268–69, 289, 291, 295–96, 351, 357
compassion, 176, 342, 353
daily activities, 92, 328
encounter, 301, 328
foot-care, 98, 327
handover report, 287
hands, 106–7, 327
interaction, 278, 328
life, 63, 361
lifting, 131, 328
medication administration, 275, 328
posture, 129, 328
reflection, 274, 328
reflective practice, 273, 361

speech, 54, 256, 328, 351

steps, 94, 327

teamwork, 249

mindfulness, 15–19, 29–34, 36–38, 43–44, 75–81, 138–42, 182, 236–38, 245–47, 306–11, 314–17, 327–28, 333–36, 338–40, 353–56

  daily, 42, 317, 323

  informal, 42, 86

  bell, 299, 304, 327, 333

  instructors, 313–14

  meditation, 336, 340, 352, 356, 367

  practice, 28, 36, 38, 41–42, 59, 65, 67, 73, 75–76, 85, 275, 314, 340, 355

    daily, 74, 86

  trainers, 314, 335

Mindfulness Bell, practice, 304

Mindfulness of Sounds, practice, 115

mistakes, 20–21, 28, 48, 58, 145, 147, 200, 205–6, 209, 224, 240, 271–76, 278, 284–85, 289

monitor, 65, 273, 299–304, 306

monkey mind, 25–26, 38–39, 64, 238

motivation, 66, 176, 179, 181, 183, 312, 346, 355

movement practice, mindful, 158–59, 161, 170

movements

  body's, 118–19

  mindful, 38, 157, 159–62, 168–70, 185, 198, 210, 269, 328, 335

muscles, 20–21, 60, 97, 111, 117, 120, 130–31, 163, 215, 231

N

negative thoughts, 76, 138, 141, 215, 224, 236

nonjudgment, 174, 179, 181–82

nurse practitioner, 73, 77, 100, 252

nurses

  cardiac, 60, 275

  charge, 177, 244

  compassionate, 174, 193, 232

  less-experienced, 253

  mindful, 77, 182, 257, 306

  outgoing, 292

  outgoing shift, 290

nurse-to-patient ratio influence, 117

Nursing Stress Scale, 15, 145, 341

nursing tasks, 146, 292

O

Observing Thoughts, practice, 238

P

pain

  acute, 138, 335

  chest, 187, 190, 277, 283

  chronic, 131, 136, 138, 335

  experiencing, 137, 287

  reduced, 175, 342, 352

  secondary, 139–40, 142

pain medication, 193

pain relief, 168, 335

pain score, patient's, 300

pain sensations, 138, 141

patient care, 36, 45, 151, 197, 225, 245, 250, 255, 297, 301, 320, 343, 363

patient complaints, 288, 299

patients

  difficult, 42, 150

  distressed, 26

  lift, 90, 106

  new, 143, 250

patient safety, 76, 254, 288–89, 295

personal life, 50, 96, 329

physicians, 146–47, 310, 321

pose, 161–67

  mountain, 165–67

posture, 83, 129–30, 133–34, 157–58, 167, 260

Q

qualities, compassionate, 181–82

R

relief nurse, 281

response, emotional, 115, 180

resting, 107, 110, 266

rhythm, patient's, 303

rumination, 152, 201, 206, 211, 236

S

self-care, 18, 21, 90–91, 96, 102, 136, 196–97, 320, 325, 334, 336
  mindful, 89, 98
self-compassion, 15, 20–21, 36, 161, 199, 201–3, 205–7, 209–11, 325
  mindful, 207
  moderate, 204
  practicing, 206, 211
Self-compassion Break, 207–8, 210, 328
self-compassion practice, 206, 209
self-compassion scores, 204
senior nurses
  compassionate, 230
  uncompassionate, 230
sensations, 30–31, 64–66, 83, 108, 110, 118–19, 122, 130, 137, 139–42, 156–57, 159–61, 167, 239, 265–66
  difficult, 140–42, 328
  unpleasant, 73, 111, 139–40, 167, 221
Short Body Scan, practice, 113
shoulders, 49, 73, 105, 111, 113–14, 120, 128–30, 140, 163–65
situations, difficult, 79, 226, 228, 259
sounds
  mindfulness of, 113–15, 239, 327
  noticing, 115–16

staff, 40, 81, 134–35, 146, 186, 221, 261, 268, 307, 310–12, 315, 317–19, 321
STOP practice, 279–80, 285, 327
stress, everyday, 13, 123, 335
stressful situations, 21, 44, 78, 154, 156, 268, 286
stress levels, 79, 145, 148, 273, 283, 286, 308, 331
stressors, 149, 151, 156, 273
stress reaction, 150–52, 155, 284
STS (secondary traumatic stress), 330–31
student nurses, 230, 232
sympathy, 175, 179–81
symptoms, 20, 95, 103, 138, 148, 158, 189, 191, 195, 197, 262, 292, 294, 330

T

tasks, 27–29, 32, 34, 40, 45–46, 48–53, 63, 65, 68–69, 84–85, 93, 249–51, 273–74, 282, 293
technology, 94, 277, 297–302, 304–6, 338, 361, 365
telemetry, 89, 199–200, 302
tension, 49, 52, 81, 83, 85, 98, 101, 109–10, 112–13, 115–16, 118, 120, 148–49, 168–69, 250
The 3Ps, practice, 54

Three-step Breathing Space, practice, 82–86, 156, 296, 327
thoughts, 25–26, 35, 39, 41, 47, 60, 73–76, 111–15, 137–39, 152, 154–57, 217–18, 235–42, 245–47, 263–66
Tonglen-on-the-spot, practice, 226–27, 328
touch, 14, 32, 47, 65, 104–6, 164, 166, 194, 261, 294, 298
traumatic stress, secondary, 330
trial, randomized controlled, 206, 346, 355, 360
trust, 36, 49, 67, 71, 77, 161, 231, 255, 267
Two Feet, One Breath, practice, 284

U

understanding, compassionate, 173, 203, 205

W

weight, 62, 64–65, 97–98, 107, 110, 118–19, 129, 131, 166–67, 241
workplace, compassionate, 317–18
worry, 21–22, 25–26, 58–61, 80, 83, 90, 120, 123, 182, 208, 213, 217, 240, 246, 319

Y

yoga, 95, 129, 157–60, 335–36, 343, 358

About the Author

Carmel Sheridan, MA, MSc, is a licensed psychotherapist and supervisor in private practice. She has two master's degrees in psychology and is author of two books: *Failure-Free Activities for the Alzheimer's Patient*, and *Reminiscence: Uncovering a Lifetime of Memories*. A long-time meditator, Carmel teaches mindfulness and compassion-based practices to healthcare professionals, including nurses, with a focus on self-compassion to promote resilience, focus, self-care, and well-being. She also teaches the eight-week Mindfulness-Based Stress Reduction program in workplaces, in the community, as well as online. Carmel regularly takes time out from teaching to attend retreats around the world. Contact her at carmel@nursingmindfully.com.

CPSIA information can be obtained
at www.ICGtesting.com
Printed in the USA
LVOW05s2318280817
546746LV00019B/489/P